Main

Weight Loss Surgery

FOR

DUMMIES®

2ND EDITION

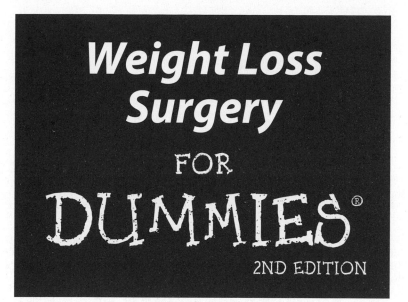

Weight Loss Surgery

FOR

DUMMIES®

2ND EDITION

by Marina S. Kurian, MD, Barbara Thompson, and Brian K. Davidson

Foreword by Al Roker
NBC Weatherman and Television Personality

WILEY

John Wiley & Sons, Inc.

Weight Loss Surgery For Dummies®, 2nd Edition

Published by
John Wiley & Sons, Inc.
111 River St.
Hoboken, NJ 07030-5774
www.wiley.com

WILEY

About the Authors

Marina S. Kurian, MD: Dr. Marina Kurian grew up in New York City and attended Stuyvesant High School. She graduated summa cum laude with a BS degree from Union College and received her MD from Albany Medical College. Dr. Kurian completed her general surgery training at Albany Medical Center in Albany, New York. She completed additional training and is board certified in both general surgery and surgical critical care. After completing an advanced laparoscopic fellowship, she started her practice in July 2000. Dr. Kurian's interest in weight loss surgery started in her general surgery training and was honed in her advanced laparoscopic fellowship. She is currently the medical director of the New York University Langone Medical Center Weight Management Program. As a recognized expert in the field of obesity surgery, she has spoken at many national and international meetings on the topic of obesity. She is the author of many articles and book chapters on laparoscopic surgery. Dr. Kurian is active in the American Society of Metabolic & Bariatric Surgery (ASMBS) and the Society of American Gastrointestinal and Endoscopic Surgeons (SAGES) and is a Fellow of the American College of Surgeons (FACS). She also is a weekly host on *Doctor Radio* (Sirius/XM 81), discussing a variety of health topics.

Barbara Thompson: Barbara Thompson is a gastric bypass patient, author, and professional speaker. She battled a weight problem from the day she was born. When she finally admitted to herself in her late 20s that her "baby fat" was turning into a serious problem, she began dieting earnestly, only to diet her way to severe obesity. Over her adult life, Barbara experienced the very common pattern of losing weight, regaining it, and adding a few additional pounds. When her weight reached 264 pounds and a herniated disk in her back was causing her to face disability, she knew she was in trouble. She decided to have the life-altering gastric bypass surgery in January 2000 at the University of Pittsburgh Medical Center.

Today, Barbara is a national speaker on weight loss surgery, obesity sensitivity, and getting control of your life. She is the author of *Weight Loss Surgery: Finding the Thin Person Hiding Inside You*. She hosts the patient website www.wlscenter.com; the Facebook group WLS Private; and her blog, www.weightlosssurgeryblog.net.

Barbara is a past chairman of the board of the Obesity Action Coalition, a member of the American Society of Metabolic and Bariatric Surgery Corporate Council, and a member of the National Speakers Association. She lives in Pittsburgh with her husband, Frank, and daughter, Erin. You can contact her through www.wlscenter.com.

Brian K. Davidson: Brian is the coauthor of *Weight Loss Surgery Cookbook For Dummies.* Brian has been featured on television, spoken at various industry events, and consulted with leading industry professionals and patients. He has authored several articles for the weight loss surgery community. He is a passionate advocate and dedicated to improving obesity awareness and increasing public education for this devastating disease. Brian lives in Connecticut and is the proud father of his daughter, Grace, and son, Riley. You can contact him at bk311d@gmail.com.

Dedication

This book is dedicated to everyone who is afflicted with the disease of severe obesity. It is dedicated to all those who have tried to diet and failed over and over again, only to find themselves gaining more and more weight. It is also dedicated to the families of those with this disease, in the hopes that they will find understanding and a way to offer support. It is our desire that you find information and hope within the covers of this book.

Authors' Acknowledgments

The authors would like to acknowledge the many people who have contributed to this book. We are grateful to Tony Augsburger, Teesha Murphy, and Cindy Phipps for their inspiring before and after pictures and success stories and to Jessica MacKechnie for the use of her bariatric food guide pyramid. We also would like to thank the following patients who contributed their thoughts, which are sprinkled throughout this book: Kalli Cagle, Sandy Fields, Amanda Foxworth, Susan Hartmann, Jackie Hutchison, Stacy Leary, Tammy St. Clair, Janet Santos, Marjorie Schuyler, and Michele Weston.

We would like to offer a special thanks to Dr. Sayeed Ikramuddin of the Center for Minimally Invasive Surgery, University of Minnesota, Minneapolis, for serving as our technical editor; to Michael Lewis of Wiley, whose belief in this project was pivotal; and to Elizabeth Kuball, freelance editor, for her editing and good counsel. Thanks also to Al Roker for being kind and generous enough to write the foreword.

The authors are indebted to David Fouts, bariatric chef and weight loss surgery patient, for submitting all the recipes for this book, which are designed to help the weight loss surgery patient not only adjust to a new way of eating but learn to enjoy a healthier way of life. David is the author of *Culinary Classics: Essentials of Cooking for the Gastric Bypass Patient*. His website is www.chefdave.org.

From Marina:

I have a personal mantra that I will share. Every day, I wake up and try to do better. Part of that means doing work at night after my "day job" is over. My family makes concessions and excuses all the time. My kids think it's great that I do all this "stuff" but would love for me to just hang out and be available to them. To my family, I say, "You make me better and in a cruel twist make me want to do more. Because you make me happy and ground me, I am able to stretch and reach for the highest branches." To my patients who have trusted me to take care of them, who continue to see me (because it really is lifelong care), who teach me about resiliency in the face of adversity, who show me there is always a way, who have lifted me on my down days, I thank you. I have immense job satisfaction because of you all. Not everyone can be so lucky.

From Barbara:

I am indebted to the thousands of patients I have met in my travels and at speaking engagements. They have inspired me beyond words with their courage and newfound love of life. And to the many surgeons and healthcare professionals who work with these patients — I have never met a more compassionate and caring group of people who love what they are doing. I am especially indebted to Dr. Phil Schauer, now at Cleveland Clinic, who performed my surgery and has remained a lifelong friend.

And to my husband, Frank. I could not do what I do if it weren't for his love, support, guidance, and patience. His chapter in my first book addressed to significant others has helped thousands of families understand what patients go through and how they can provide loving support. And to the delight of my life, my daughter, Erin. I bless the day that she came into my life.

From Brian:

I would like to give a special thanks to my parents, Myrna and Bob. To my children, Grace and Riley, who inspire me with the beauty of their spirit, compassion, joy, and love. To all those who have helped me along this wonderful journey, thanks from the bottom of my heart.

Publisher's Acknowledgments

We're proud of this book; please send us your comments through our Dummies online registration form located at www.dummies.com/register/.

Some of the people who helped bring this book to market include the following:

Acquisitions and Editorial

Project Editor: Elizabeth Kuball
  (Previous Edition: Elizabeth Kuball)

Acquisitions Editor: Michael Lewis

Copy Editor: Elizabeth Kuball
  (Previous Edition: Elizabeth Kuball)

Assistant Editor: David Lutton

Editorial Program Coordinator: Joe Niesen

Technical Editor: Sayeed Ikramuddin, MD

Senior Editorial Manager: Jennifer Ehrlich

Editorial Manager: Carmen Krikorian

Editorial Assistants: Rachelle S. Amick,
  Alexa Koschier

Art Coordinator: Alicia B. South

Cover Photos: © iStockPhoto.com/Andi Berger

Cartoons: Rich Tennant
  (www.the5thwave.com)

Composition Services

Sr. Project Coordinator: Kristie Rees

Layout and Graphics: Jennifer Creasey,
  Lavonne Roberts

Proofreaders: Lindsay Amones,
  BIM Indexing & Proofreading Services

Indexer: BIM Indexing & Proofreading Services

Illustrator: Kathryn Born

Recipe Tester: Emily Nolan

Nutrition Analyst: Patricia Santelli

Publishing and Editorial for Consumer Dummies

  Kathleen Nebenhaus, Vice President and Executive Publisher

  David Palmer, Associate Publisher

  Kristin Ferguson-Wagstaffe, Product Development Director

Publishing for Technology Dummies

  Andy Cummings, Vice President and Publisher

Composition Services

  Debbie Stailey, Director of Composition Services

Contents at a Glance

Recipes at a Glance

Seafood

Shakes

Table of Contents

Foreword

I sometimes tell people that Dr. Marina Kurian gave me my life back. I have struggled with my weight my entire adult life. I dieted my way to a low of 185 pounds in the mid 1970s and went up and down through the –'80s and –'90s till I topped out at 325 pounds during the 2002 Winter Olympics. By then I had decided to have gastric bypass surgery and was scheduled for the procedure with Dr. K., as I like to call her, in March 2002.

It wasn't a decision I made lightly. I researched the procedure on the Internet, I spoke with bypass patients, and I interviewed eight different doctors before I came to make this choice.

My surgery has been a great success, but one that comes with a price. This book is a great help to those who are considering the surgery, as well as their family and friends. It explains the various procedures, the risks, the possible complications, and what goes on after you've started losing weight. I wish it had been out when I had my surgery.

I have always been very careful when talking about the surgery. I have never endorsed it, and in only a couple of cases have I ever recommended it. I do, however, recommend this book, only because of the people who are behind it.

Weight Loss Surgery For Dummies is really for smart people who want to make an intelligent, informed choice.

Al Roker
NBC Weatherman and Television Personality
New York, New York

Introduction

● ●

You've probably heard a lot about weight loss surgery in the media, with celebrities going public about their stories. Reporters may have used words like *extreme* or *dangerous* to describe the surgery. Maybe you were online and saw before and after pictures of a patient. The pictures were motivating, and you thought, "Wouldn't it be nice to be the after picture for a change?"

But those pictures leave a lot of questions unanswered. How did the patients do it? How did they decide what procedure or surgeon was best for them? Did they have any struggles or complications? How long have they kept the weight off? What was their secret?

Answering those questions is what *Weight Loss Surgery For Dummies,* 2nd Edition, is about. In this book, you'll find the truth about weight loss surgery. We take the mystery out of deciding whether the operation is right for you, and we show you how to become that person in the after picture.

About This Book

Weight loss surgery is not a magic potion that miraculously takes off the pounds forever. Although it may be the right choice for some, it isn't for everyone. Weight loss surgery is a life-changing procedure, so if you're thinking about going through it, you should have a solid understanding of what will take place and what you'll need to do to live well after the procedure. Before you head into the operating room, you also should be aware of complications that may occur after your surgery. Your surgeon will provide you with a tool — your surgery — to assist you in leading a slimmer and healthier life. Making that tool work through behavior modifications, a healthy eating plan, exercise, and emotional support is up to you. This book empowers you to make the best choice for you.

Conventions Used in This Book

Here's an overview of the conventions we use in this book:

- ✔ Occasionally we use technical or medical terms that you may not be familiar with. Any new terms are *italicized* and are followed with an explanation in parentheses.

- ✔ E-mail and web addresses appear in `monofont`, so you can easily spot them. ***Note:*** When this book was printed, some web addresses may have needed to break across two lines of text. If that happened, rest assured that we haven't put in any extra characters (such as hyphens) to indicate the break. So, when using one of these web addresses, just type in exactly what you see in this book, pretending as though the line break doesn't exist.

- ✔ All vegetarian recipes (recipes without meat) are flagged with a ☺.

In this second edition of the book, we use the term *severe obesity* instead of *morbid obesity*. Both terms have been used interchangeably for years, but the term *morbid obesity* carries more of a negative bias, so we've opted not to use it here.

Foolish Assumptions

If you're interested in this book, we've made a few assumptions about you:

- ✔ You or someone you love suffers from severe obesity and related physical complications.

- ✔ You're interested in finding out more about weight loss surgery and whether it's the right choice for you.

- ✔ You've tried to lose weight through diets, exercise, popular weight loss programs, and perhaps even diet drugs — all to no avail. You've felt shame and despair after each failed attempt.

- ✔ You've already had weight loss surgery and you're looking for a resource to maintain your weight loss and successfully manage all the post-op challenges.

- ✔ Being obese has posed serious social, family, or lifestyle obstacles and has become central to your identity.

- ✔ You're tired of sitting back and watching life pass you by. You're ready to reach out and grab life by the horns.

- ✔ You're looking for a permanent solution for your weight problem and a healthier future.

How This Book Is Organized

Weight Loss Surgery For Dummies is divided into six parts. The material is organized so you don't have to start at the beginning. If you prefer, you can turn directly to the chapter that contains the information you need. Here's a rundown of what you'll find in each part.

Part 1: Is Weight Loss Surgery for You?

This part details the different types of weight loss surgery procedures, how they work to help you lose weight, and the pros and cons of each. We also discuss the criteria your surgeon will use to determine if you're a candidate for surgery. Understanding all there is to know about this lifelong commitment is vitally important. You need to know what can go wrong with surgery, so your decision is an informed one. You also need to find and work with healthcare professionals you can trust. In this part, we arm you with a list of questions and criteria to help you find the best possible surgeon and healthcare team for you.

Part II: Preparing for Surgery

After you've determined that weight loss surgery is right for you, this part explains what to expect before surgery. Will your insurance cover the procedure? If so, how much does your insurance pay and how much will you have to pay yourself? What options do you have if your insurance refuses to pay? We provide you with detailed information regarding paying for surgery. We also tell you about tests you'll be required to take prior to surgery and the reasons behind these tests.

To be as safe as possible during surgery and to help prepare for the changes after surgery, you need to be physically ready. Starting to lose weight now, by moderately exercising and changing your eating habits, is a good idea. In this part, we provide suggestions on how to do that.

Part III: The Hospital Experience and Beyond

The big transition begins now. This part takes you from what to expect while you're in the hospital to your initial experiences after surgery. Your eating guidelines after surgery will start with only liquids and progress to soft foods and eventually back to regular chow. You'll also find delicious recipes that are appropriate for each stage. We also show you how to field questions about your surgery when you go back to work and discuss the importance of enlisting the help of family and friends.

Part IV: This Time I'm Going to Make It: Ensuring Success

You may not be at your ideal weight, but are you a success or a failure? In this part, we look at what determines success. We also detail how to lose the weight and keep it off for life through a healthy eating plan and exercise. Weight loss and maintenance are difficult, and you won't want to go it alone. In this part, we suggest ways you can get the emotional and physical support you need.

Part V: Changing Outside and In

Most people would agree that dealing with the changes after surgery are much more difficult than the actual hospital stay and recovery. You may experience unpleasant side effects such as nausea, dumping, and hair loss. You also may have some emotional issues such as head hunger, depression, and trying to cope with stress without eating. In this part, we discuss physical and emotional challenges and how to overcome them. We also detail changes in your personal relationships and provide guidance to those who are considering plastic surgery.

Part VI: The Part of Tens

A mainstay of all *For Dummies* books is the Part of Tens. Here you'll find lists of weight loss surgery benefits, myths and misconceptions about weight loss surgery, and ways to stay on the straight and narrow.

Icons Used in This Book

Icons are those little pictures you see in the margins of the book. We've put them there to draw your attention to particular kinds of information:

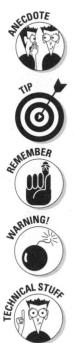

When you see the Dummies Man whispering in someone's ear, you can bet you'll find someone's personal story to inspire you in your weight loss surgery journey.

This icon points you to a good idea that will help you achieve your goals.

When we flag text with this icon, you can bet it's important information that's worth remembering.

This icon points out some common mistakes that you should avoid or other dangers along the way.

When the discussion becomes a little too technical, you'll see this icon. You can skip over anything marked with a Technical Stuff icon, but if you're looking to impress your surgeon the next time you talk, look no further.

Where to Go from Here

If you're considering surgery, you can start with Chapter 1 and read the book from beginning to end. If you have specific questions that you want answers to now, feel free to skip around as you see fit. For example, to find the right surgeon for you, check out Chapter 5. If you want to know if you qualify for surgery, check out Chapter 2. If you have a surgery scheduled, you may want to start with Chapter 7, which familiarizes you with the various testing procedures you'll be required to have before surgery. You'll also find important information on how to prepare for surgery in Chapter 8.

If you've already had surgery, you'll find valuable information that addresses common issues in whatever stage you're in. If you recently had surgery, you may want to start with Chapter 10. If you're looking for delicious and healthy recipes, turn to Chapters 10, 11, and 15.

Wherever you start, we wish you luck on your weight loss surgery journey!

Part I

Is Weight Loss Surgery for You?

The 5th Wave   By Rich Tennant

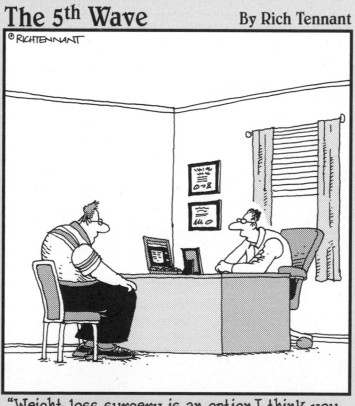

"Weight loss surgery is an option I think you should keep on your plate, so to speak."

In this part . . .

You've probably heard about weight loss surgery, but is it really for you? In this part, you find out. We tell you what it takes to qualify for surgery and help you examine if you're ready to make the necessary lifelong commitment to a healthier lifestyle. Being successful with weight loss surgery takes more than an operation, and we detail what is necessary to reach and maintain your goal weight.

There is not just one type of operation for weight loss surgery. In this part, you discover all the different surgeries available and how they work to promote weight loss. You also find out about the pros and cons of each surgery, as well as the risks involved.

The task of selecting a surgeon is an important one, and in this part we give you questions to ask and criteria with which to make an informed choice. Part of the consideration is evaluating your surgeon's team. There are support members of the surgical practice whose job it is to help you be as successful as you can be. In this part, you discover the role each person plays in that accomplishment.

Chapter 1

The Ins and Outs of Weight Loss Surgery

In This Chapter

▶ Understanding how weight loss surgery works

▶ Deciding whether surgery is right for you

▶ Preparing for and dealing with the lifestyle changes

*M*aking the decision to have weight loss surgery is a major commitment to your overall health. It's usually the last resort after years of struggling and trying other methods to lose weight and live a healthier life. Weight loss surgery, also known as *bariatric surgery,* is currently the only treatment available that has been found to be effective as a long-term treatment for severe obesity. The results after surgery are, for the most part, extraordinary, not only in terms of appearance but also in terms of the improvement in or removal of health risks associated with obesity.

If you're considering weight loss surgery, being well informed about the procedure and how your life will change following surgery is essential. The procedure itself is only a tool to assist you in losing weight and modifying your behavior. Success is up to you. After weight loss surgery, you have to be careful about choosing foods wisely, taking your vitamins and supplements regularly, making exercise a part of your daily life, and being certain to follow your doctor's directions. You'll need a support system of family and friends to get through the emotional and physical ups and downs.

With any surgery, risks are involved. Before you decide to have weight loss surgery, you need to understand — and accept — the risks and benefits. For many patients, the risk of death from *not* having the weight loss surgery is greater than the risks of having the procedure itself.

There's no place like thin

My story starts out like many others who suffer from the disease of obesity. I battled a weight problem from the day I was born. When I finally admitted to myself in my late 20s that my "baby fat" was turning into a serious problem, I began dieting earnestly, only to diet my way to severe obesity.

Over my adult life, I experienced the very common pattern of losing weight, regaining it, and adding a few additional pounds. This cycle continued many times. When my weight reached 264 pounds, and a herniated disk in my back was causing me to face disability, I knew I was in trouble. Although I didn't have the many health problems associated with obesity — such as heart disease, high blood pressure, or diabetes — I felt it was only a matter of time before I would develop them.

I decided to have gastric bypass surgery in January 2000. At that time, there were no books on weight loss surgery, so everything I found out about the surgery came from my own research of medical journals and from other patients.

My recovery from the surgery was fairly routine, even though it was long. The surgery was harder on me than I expected, and it was eight weeks before I felt like I had a spring in my step. I watched as others having the surgery bounced back in two weeks and I was still limping along. That taught me that each person is different in her response to the surgery. The support of my husband after my surgery was very important. My recovery would have been very different were it not for his love and understanding.

My weight loss was slower than many of those I knew, and that worried me. But what I found is that everyone loses at his own pace, and the rate of loss is not always a gauge of how much weight a patient ultimately loses.

Throughout my weight loss journey I have tried to follow four basic principles:

✔ At meals, I eat my protein first.

✔ I try my best not to graze on foods throughout the day.

✔ Water is more important than most people realize, so I strive for 64 ounces per day.

✔ I exercise — probably the most important yet the most difficult for me!

In 18 months, I went from facing disability to completing a 22-mile bike ride after losing 125 pounds. But as thrilling as that day was, it was just as thrilling the day I stood at the bottom of my stairs and ran to the top and didn't think I was going to die! Being able to do the ordinary things are just as wondrous as the extraordinary things. Being able to tie my shoes, paint my toenails, take a bath (and have water on both sides of me), and shop, shop, shop are a regained blessing. And having this chance to live and thrive is something I don't take for granted. I've been able to reach for a whole new life as an author and a national speaker, something I never would have had the self-esteem to do before my surgery. I am grateful that I found my solution.

Barbara Thompson
Patient, speaker, and author

Is Weight Loss Surgery Right for You?

For people who are severely obese, trying to lose weight without surgery isn't as effective when it comes to achieving significant long-term weight loss.

The majority of severely obese people who try to lose weight without having weight loss surgery regain all the weight they've lost over the next five years. Surgical treatment is the only proven method of achieving long-term significant weight control.

So, how do you know if you're severely obese? In general, individuals are considered severely obese if their weight is more than 100 pounds over their ideal body weight. But a more common way to define severe obesity is to use the body mass index (BMI). These days, you can't go online without stumbling over a BMI calculator. This is a quick way to check your level of obesity.

In Chapter 2, we also provide a chart to help you figure out your BMI. If your BMI puts you in the severely obese category, you may be a candidate for weight loss surgery. If your weight is lower, but you have other health problems related to obesity; if you've tried to lose weight and failed; and if you're aware of all the risks and rewards of weight loss surgery, weight loss surgery may be the solution for you.

How Does the Surgery Work?

Several types of procedures to achieve weight loss are being done today. These procedures can be divided into three basic categories:

- ✔ **Restrictive procedures,** which limit the amount of food you can eat
- ✔ **Malabsorptive procedures,** which alter your normal digestive process, causing food to be poorly digested and only partially absorbed
- ✔ **A combination of restrictive and malabsorptive**

With restrictive procedures, like gastric banding, the size of the stomach is reduced by sectioning the stomach with a band. The smaller pouch above the band usually holds no more than 1 to 3 ounces of food, which causes the feeling of fullness after just a few bites. The intestines continue to function normally to absorb nutrients.

Another restrictive procedure is the sleeve gastrectomy, in which part of the stomach is completely removed from the body. Your stomach is made to hold approximately 2 to 3 ounces of food at a meal, so you eat a lot less. Another benefit of the sleeve gastrectomy: The part of the stomach that is removed makes a hormone that makes you hungry, so when that part of the stomach is gone, most sleeve gastrectomy patients are much less hungry.

A gastric bypass procedure combines restriction and malabsorption by limiting the amount of food that can be consumed and limiting the amount of time that this food can be absorbed by the body. In gastric bypass, the surgeon makes a small pouch from the stomach, bypassing most of the stomach and a part of the small intestines. The small gastric pouch usually holds about 1 ounce of food. The small intestines are reattached to the new smaller pouch. Operations that cause malabsorption and restrict food intake typically produce more weight loss than restrictive procedures, which only decrease food intake.

A malabsorptive procedure like the duodenal switch bypasses most of the small intestines so that much of what you eat is not absorbed. A malabsorptive procedure will result in a greater weight loss but carries with it the greatest possibility of complications and nutritional deficiencies.

In addition to the type of surgery you choose, other factors that influence weight loss are

- ✔ **Your age:** As you age, your metabolism slows. The older you are, the more slowly you'll lose weight. Women also get the double whammy of menopause, which slows the metabolism further.

- ✔ **Your sex:** Because men have a higher percentage of muscle than women, men burn fat and lose weight faster than women.

- ✔ **Your ethnicity:** Some studies suggest that African-American women don't lose as much weight as their Caucasian counterparts. But even with less weight loss, the health improvements are the same.

- ✔ **Your weight at the time of the surgery:** Patients who are severely over-weight have more to lose and, as a result, drop more pounds. But they may not get as close to their ideal body weight.

What Are the Risks and Benefits?

The most apparent benefit of weight loss surgery is the sometimes rapid and more-often-than-not permanent weight loss. Less visible but probably most important are the health improvements that occur from losing the weight. The surgery has been found to be effective in improving and controlling many obesity-related health conditions, including the following:

- ✔ Diabetes
- ✔ High blood pressure
- ✔ Sleep apnea
- ✔ Osteoarthritis
- ✔ Symptoms of gastroesophageal reflux disease (GERD)
- ✔ Infertility

- ✔ Heart disease
- ✔ Respiratory problems
- ✔ High cholesterol and triglycerides
- ✔ Cardiovascular function

Other benefits include more energy and improved self-esteem, as well as improved mobility and comfort.

As with any surgery, however, weight loss surgery is associated with some long-term complications and risks. Risk of death from complications of surgery is less than 1 percent. Depending upon the type of procedure, other possible risks include (but are not limited to) the following:

- ✔ Bleeding
- ✔ Bowel obstruction
- ✔ Cardiac problems
- ✔ Complications due to anesthesia and medications
- ✔ Deep vein thrombosis (DVT)
- ✔ Pulmonary embolus
- ✔ *Dehiscence* (problems with muscle healing)
- ✔ Dehydration
- ✔ *Dumping syndrome* (an adverse reaction to eating foods high in fat and sugar; see Chapter 18)
- ✔ *Esophageal dilation* (an enlargement of the diameter of the esophagus to greater-than-normal size)
- ✔ *Gastric prolapse* (a slippage of the stomach around an adjustable band)
- ✔ Gastrointestinal leaks
- ✔ Hernia
- ✔ Infection
- ✔ Iron and vitamin deficiencies
- ✔ *Stricture* (a narrowing of the intestines)
- ✔ Ulcers

Chapter 4 covers the risks of surgery in more detail. But remember: Only you and your doctor can determine whether weight loss surgery is right for you.

Not the easy way out

The majority of the general public is misinformed about obesity and weight loss surgery. They still think that severe obesity is a disease of willpower; that if you would just eat less, you would lose weight; that somehow you let yourself go. They don't know that it is a disease of genes and hormones or that needing to lose 5 pounds is a lot different from needing to lose 100 pounds.

If you're obese, you know what you've been through. Most people have no idea what it's like for you to struggle with obesity — how obesity-related physical problems have affected your daily life; the mental anguish of being treated differently because of your weight and how this destroys your self-esteem; how obesity interferes with all aspects of your life and the never-ending frustration of trying to overcome it.

They also have no understanding of the countless diets you've tried and that, even though you may have lost some weight on those diets, the weight always returned, sometimes with some unwelcome extra pounds. They don't know that the exercise, commercial weight loss programs, and prescription pills you've tried have failed again and again. They also don't know about the countless hours you've spent researching and investigating this surgery.

You've probably struggled to get insurance coverage, undergone all kinds of medical tests, and endured pain, nausea, and other unpleasant side effects from your surgery. The fact that you've had to change your eating habits and exercise routine also are not accounted for. Having friends, family, and even people who wouldn't talk to you before your surgery treating you differently is also a difficult adjustment. This is all in addition to the emotional and psychological changes you're experiencing.

So, the next time someone tells you weight loss surgery is the easy way out, you can tell them exactly how "easy" it is.

Which Surgeon Should You Go To?

The surgeon is the head of your team and will be the team's most important member. You'll want to find an experienced and dedicated surgeon who offers a comprehensive weight loss surgery program — including support personnel and programs to help you with the best preparation before and follow-up care after surgery.

Make sure your surgeon is a Center of Excellence surgeon. The American Society for Metabolic & Bariatric Surgery and the American College of Surgeons have designated certain bariatric programs, based on multiple stringent criteria, as Center of Excellence programs. Certain insurance companies also evaluate bariatric programs and give them a center of excellence designation. What all this really means is that the program and the surgeon are experienced, have been closely vetted, and meet some high standards. It also means that your surgeon keeps track of how well she and her patients are doing. You should be able to ask all the important questions and get the answers at your visit with her. (Choosing a surgeon is such an important undertaking that we devote Chapter 5 to the topic.)

The way to find your perfect fit is to shop around. You can get a good feel for a practice by visiting and asking questions. Call the office and ask if it runs meetings where you can find out more about the surgery. You can get a feel for how the surgeon and his support staff treat you, and you can find answers to your specific questions. Attend not only the informational meetings but support-group meetings as well, because support groups are a vital part of your recovery.

Will Your Surgery Be Covered by Insurance?

The actual process of convincing your insurance company to pay for the procedure may be just as difficult and almost as much work as the procedure itself. Although most insurance companies do pay for weight loss surgery, it sometimes requires a lengthy and complicated approval process. Each company has its own authorization requirements.

Start by calling your insurance carrier and asking if your policy has coverage for weight loss surgery. If your policy excludes coverage for obesity or weight loss, this is different from excluding coverage for severe obesity — so your policy may still cover weight loss surgery. Some employers have purchased insurance plans that don't cover weight loss surgery because it's cheaper for their company. You may want to reach out to your human resources representative and see if it's possible for the company to upgrade your policy to include weight loss surgery.

Be sure you understand the specifics of your policy and what's required to obtain approval. Most companies require a letter of medical necessity from your obesity surgeon and your primary-care physician. Many carriers also require a nutritional consult and psychological evaluation. Some may refer you to a doctor-supervised diet program of several months' duration before granting approval.

Don't take the first "no" as an answer. Many patients are covered following an appeal.

For more information on insurance, turn to Chapter 6.

What Lifestyle Changes Will You Have to Make?

In order to make the most of your weight loss surgery, you'll need to modify your lifestyle after the surgery. Here are some changes you'll need to make:

✔ **You'll need to restrict your diet and take supplements.** Because the size of your stomach has effectively been reduced to about the size of 1 cup or less, your meals will be in smaller portions. You'll need to make sure you chew your food slowly and thoroughly, so it doesn't become stuck and so it's properly digested. You'll need more time to eat than you used to, but you'll also notice you feel fuller with less food. You won't drink any beverages with your meal — your stomach will be too small to hold both. If you had gastric bypass or duodenal switch surgery, you'll be absorbing fewer nutrients than you did before the surgery, so to prevent deficiencies, you'll need to commit to a regimen of vitamin supplements for the rest of your life. It's a good idea for gastric banding and sleeve gastrectomy patients to take a multivitamin as well. (Turn to Chapters 10, 11, and 15 for much more information on food, including some great recipes to try every step of the way.)

✔ **You'll need to exercise regularly.** You're probably already aware of the benefits of exercise to your overall health and well-being. Exercise is even more important to the weight loss surgery patient. After surgery, you'll be losing weight rapidly. When this happens, your body will burn stored fat and muscle. Exercising and eating more protein are important in countering this by building muscle, burning fat, and increasing your metabolism. Exercise also will be crucial in helping you maintain your weight loss and healthy lifestyle for the long term. (Chapter 16 offers more information on getting into the routine of regular exercise.)

✔ **You'll need to work through any psychological and emotional issues.** Many people mistakenly assume that weight loss surgery will be a quick fix to all their problems. You have your own issues going into the surgery, and chances are, you'll still have some of them after surgery. Weight loss surgery will affect most aspects of your life, including your family, career, social life, and self-esteem. You'll be faced with a lot of changes, most of them good. But any change — good or bad — causes some degree of stress and anxiety. Consider this as possibly added stress to the issues you already have. Recognize that food has been part of your coping mechanism. As you go through the weight loss journey, it's important to find a different coping mechanism. Participating in a support group or getting professional help through counseling will be helpful in overcoming the many challenges that you'll experience along your journey. (Chapter 19 gives you more information on these and other issues you may face after surgery.)

What New and Exciting Experiences Will You Have?

In addition to the health benefits discussed earlier in this chapter, many people find that weight loss surgery has provided them with a tool to improving their overall quality of life. This is a wonderful and motivating gift that will help keep you on track and allow you to experience new and exciting adventures. The following are only a few of the many things you can look forward to:

- Being able to enjoy life without food being a major focus
- Feeling good about yourself
- Having more energy
- Enjoying a personal freedom from being trapped and limited by your body
- Becoming more active in the lives of your children and grandchildren
- Shopping for regular-size clothes
- Crossing your legs
- Walking up stairs without being short of breath
- Walking down stairs and being able to see the steps in front of you
- Getting off your medications
- Fitting in an airplane seat, theater seat, or restaurant booth

Chapter 2

Voting for Surgery: Are You a Candidate?

In This Chapter

▶ Identifying the requirements for weight loss surgery

▶ Figuring out whether you meet the requirements

▶ Considering whether you're ready for weight loss surgery

Weight loss surgery, though it's much more common today than it was at any time in the past, is still major surgery. And as with any kind of surgery, it's not the right choice for everyone. In this chapter, we introduce you to the basic criteria that qualify patients for weight loss surgery and also fill you in on some of the additional requirements that vary from one surgeon to the next.

Weight loss surgery is a life-altering experience, one you don't want to pursue without a lot of thought and careful consultation with your doctor. You need to personally weigh the potential benefits versus the surgical risks. Usually, weight loss surgery is the last resort — after you've pursued many other options and failed.

Use this chapter to get a sense of whether you're a good fit for weight loss surgery and to prepare for your first conversation with a bariatric surgeon. Armed with the information in this chapter, you'll be able to talk with any bariatric surgeon about how your health is impacted by your weight, your dieting history, and the risks and complications you may experience.

Knowing Whether You Meet the Criteria

Weight loss surgery has been performed since the 1950s. In 1991, the National Institutes of Health (NIH) set criteria for who qualifies for the surgery and who doesn't. According to the NIH, to be a candidate for weight loss surgery, you must fit the following criteria:

- A body mass index (BMI) of 40 or above *or* a BMI of 35 or above with other *comorbidities* (health problems that are caused or made worse by excess weight)
- Failed attempts at dieting
- Knowledge of the risks and benefits of surgery

You can go to `http://consensus.nih.gov/cons/084/084_statement.htm` to read the NIH's 1991 Consensus Statement on Gastrointestinal Surgery for Severe Obesity in its entirety.

Some surgeons set additional restrictions beyond the NIH guidelines. For example, many practices will not operate on patients who are not mobile. Being mobile is very important to reduce the risk of blood clots to the lungs and pneumonia. Without mobility, the risk you face when having weight loss surgery is much higher. Therefore, if you're completely wheelchair-bound, you may be denied. Other surgeons have an age limit of 60 or 65 years. Still others won't operate on patients who have a BMI over 50. In other words, even if you meet the NIH criteria and even if you're approved by your insurance company, you still may be denied by a surgeon.

On the other hand, some surgical practices will offer weight loss surgery to lower-BMI patients, including patients with a BMI of 30 to 35 with comorbid conditions or a BMI of 35 and over without comorbid conditions.

If you don't meet the criteria set by a particular surgeon, don't try to talk him into accepting you. The surgeon has set those criteria because he's comfortable with them. Your particular health situation may present the surgeon with challenges that are beyond his expertise. If you're denied by a particular surgeon, you're much better off finding a practice that will accept you.

Ask the surgeon who's denied you if he has a recommendation for another surgeon who may be able to work with you. Surgeons generally know which of their fellow surgeons in your area have the most experience — and you want someone with a lot of experience, because your safety is dependent on it.

Measuring Your Body Mass Index

BMI is a measure that was developed to help pinpoint the height and weight at which people are more likely to have weight-related illnesses. In the past, health professionals used height and weight charts put out by life insurance companies. The Metropolitan Life Insurance Height/Weight Chart, for example, helped healthcare professionals and insurance companies predict at what weight people are more likely to die. The BMI chart helps healthcare professionals (and you!) know the weight at which you may begin to have health problems. Your surgeon will use your BMI to help determine whether you're a good candidate for weight loss surgery.

BMI is not a perfect measure of fitness. It doesn't take into consideration how much body fat you have and how your body fat is distributed. But it's the best measure available for the weight at which a person is likely to face weight-related health problems.

So, how do you find out what your BMI is? To determine your BMI, turn to Table 2-1, locate your height in inches, and then move across that row until you find your weight. The number at the top of that column is your BMI.

Measure your height before you calculate your BMI. People do shrink as they age, and obesity can compress the spine, which can affect your height. Be sure to start with a current measurement of your height. Then weigh yourself and find your height and weight on the BMI chart.

You also can go to www.nhlbisupport.com/bmi to calculate your BMI. Just enter your height and weight, and you can find your BMI. The NIH's National Heart, Lung, and Blood Institute, which provides this online calculator, even has a free iPhone app that allows you to calculate your BMI.

So, what does your BMI mean? Table 2-2 gives you the lowdown. (Turn to "Comorbidities: Identifying the Conditions Affected by Your Weight," later in this chapter, for more detailed information.)

Table 2-1

Body Mass Index

Height (inches) / BMI	35	36	37	38	39	40	41	42	43	44	45	46	47	48	49	50	51	52	53	54	55	56	57	58	59	60
	Body Weight (pounds)																									
58	167	172	177	181	186	191	196	201	205	210	215	220	224	229	234	239	244	248	253	258	263	268	273	278	283	287
59	173	178	183	188	193	198	203	208	212	217	222	227	232	237	242	247	252	257	262	267	272	277	282	287	292	297
60	179	184	189	194	199	204	209	215	220	225	230	235	240	245	250	255	261	266	271	276	282	287	292	297	302	307
61	185	190	195	201	206	211	217	222	227	232	238	243	248	254	259	264	269	275	280	285	291	296	302	307	312	318
62	191	196	202	207	213	218	224	229	235	240	246	251	256	262	267	273	278	284	289	295	301	306	312	317	323	328
63	197	203	208	214	220	225	231	237	242	248	254	259	265	270	278	282	287	293	299	304	311	316	322	327	333	339
64	204	209	215	221	227	232	238	244	250	256	262	267	273	279	285	291	296	302	308	314	321	326	332	338	344	350
65	210	216	222	228	234	240	246	252	258	264	270	276	282	288	294	300	306	312	318	324	331	337	343	349	355	361
66	216	223	229	235	241	247	253	260	266	272	278	284	291	297	303	309	315	322	328	334	341	347	353	359	366	372
67	223	230	236	242	249	255	261	268	274	280	287	293	299	306	312	319	325	331	338	344	351	358	364	370	377	383
68	230	236	243	249	256	262	269	276	282	289	295	302	308	315	322	328	335	341	348	354	362	368	375	382	388	395
69	236	243	250	257	263	270	277	284	291	297	304	311	318	324	331	338	345	351	358	365	373	379	386	393	400	406
70	243	250	257	264	271	278	285	292	299	306	313	320	327	334	341	348	355	362	369	376	383	390	397	404	411	418
71	250	257	265	272	279	286	293	301	308	315	322	329	336	343	351	358	365	372	379	386	395	402	409	416	423	430
72	258	265	272	279	287	294	302	309	316	324	331	338	346	353	361	368	375	383	390	397	406	413	421	428	435	443
73	265	272	280	288	295	302	310	318	325	333	340	348	355	363	371	378	386	393	401	408	417	425	432	440	447	455
74	272	280	287	295	303	311	319	326	334	342	350	358	365	373	381	389	396	404	412	420	428	436	444	452	460	467
75	279	287	295	303	311	319	327	335	343	351	359	367	375	383	391	399	407	415	423	431	440	448	456	464	472	480
76	287	295	304	312	320	328	336	344	353	361	369	377	385	394	402	410	418	426	435	443	452	460	468	477	485	493

Table 2-2	Understanding Your Body Mass Index
BMI	Weight Status
18.9 or below	Underweight
19 to 24.9	Normal
25 to 29.9	Overweight
30 to 34.9	Obese
35 to 49.9	Severely obese
50 or above	Super severely obese

Severe obesity is a clinical term. It isn't a value judgment, and it doesn't mean you're a bad or weak person. If your BMI puts you in the severely obese category, your chances of having significant health problems are increased. So, identifying the reality of what your weight means, and then taking positive steps to do something about it, is important.

Documenting Your Dieting History

Hundreds of weight loss diets are available, and you probably know about and have tried most of them. In fact, most people who are severely obese have gone from diet to diet searching for the answer to their weight problem. You may have gone from healthy diets (such as Weight Watchers or the Mayo Clinic Diet) to less-than-healthy diets (such as the pineapple diet or the vinegar diet). In between, you may have spent a fortune on diet programs that come with packaged foods.

You may very well have lost weight on these diets and considered yourself successful — at least for a while. And then the pounds started to creep back until you were as heavy as, or even heavier than, you were when you started. This vicious yo-yo cycle of weight loss and weight gain is not only very hard on your body but also detrimental to your self-esteem.

Now is the time for some soul searching. Have you really tried dieting? What may sound like an obvious question is an opportunity for you to examine your own dieting pattern. Consider the following:

✔ Have you been able to stay on a diet longer than a week or two?

✔ Have you discussed dieting with your primary-care physician?

✔ When dieting, have you been able to incorporate an exercise program?

If you answer "no" to any of these questions, you may want to take this opportunity to give dieting one last try. Even if you fail one more time, at least you'll know that you really did give healthy dieting a try. And remember, the motivation to avoid surgery may be what you need to stay on track this time.

If you go ahead with your plans to pursue weight loss surgery, you'll have to document your dieting pattern. Because the NIH has said that failing at dieting is one of the criteria you must meet in order to have weight loss surgery, you'll have to be able to document those failed attempts. This documentation can take many forms — be sure to check what your own insurance plan considers an official diet. Here are some examples:

- **Medically supervised diet:** This is a diet that is given to you by your primary-care physician. It may or may not include medication. It will be a sensible, balanced diet designed for you to lose a pound or two per week. With this diet, you check in with your physician at least monthly. Your doctor will document your weight, blood pressure, type of diet, and exercise plan.

- **Insurance-supervised diet:** Some insurance plans have their own weight loss programs. These programs are similar to diets supervised by physicians, but they're run by the insurance companies. Often, an insurance-supervised diet includes more psychological and social support than what you would receive through your primary-care physician.

- **Logs of commercial diets:** Weight Watchers books or logs of other commercial weight loss programs sometimes are acceptable to insurance companies. Check with your insurance company and, if this type of log is acceptable, start to put one together.

- **Personal log:** Re-creating all the diets you've been on may be a huge undertaking, but you can do it. If your insurance company will accept a personal log as proof of your dieting attempts, just take some time to go through photographs that may jog your memory and remind you of when you were larger or smaller. Check with your doctor's office to get a list of how much you weighed at each of your visits over the last five years.

If you think you may consider weight loss surgery in the future, get on a medically supervised diet immediately. Many insurance companies require that you be on a medically supervised diet for a certain period of time — some require up to six months. Some will want to see a two- to five-year history of your weight from your physician. Check with your insurance plan to see what it requires.

Comorbidities: Identifying the Conditions Affected by Your Weight

Comorbidities are health problems that are caused or made worse by excess weight. Being severely obese definitely takes its toll on the body. According to NIH guidelines, in order to be eligible for weight loss surgery, you have to have a BMI of 40 or above or a BMI of 35 or above along with comorbidities. In this section, we give you a look at the health problems that tend to go hand-in-hand with severe obesity. Understanding how your health may be affected by your weight is important in determining whether weight loss surgery is a good option for you.

When the NIH guidelines state that you must have a BMI of 40 or above or a BMI of 35 or above along with severe health problems in order to be eligible for weight loss surgery, that's a recognition of the toll that weight plays on health. Table 2-3 outlines the increased risk associated with health problems in addition to obesity.

Table 2-3	Health Risks in Relation to BMI		
BMI	*Obesity Category*	*Health Risk without Medical Problems*	*Health Risk with Medical Problems*
18.9 or below	Underweight	Slight	Minimal
19 to 24.9	Normal	None	Minimal
25 to 29.9	Overweight	Minimal	Moderate
30 to 34.9	Obese	Moderate	High
35 to 39.9	Severely obese	High	Very high
40 to 49.9	Severely obese	Very high	Extreme
50 or above	Super severely obese	Extreme	Very extreme

Heart disease

The heart is a muscle just like any other muscle in your body. The more a muscle works, the firmer and thicker it gets. For most muscles, this is a good thing — but with the heart, it is not.

The heart pumps blood at a certain rate so blood and oxygen go to all parts of the body. The larger your body is, the more your heart has to pump in order to accommodate all the distance the blood must circulate. Over time, as the heart pumps harder, the walls of the heart become thicker. This condition is called *left ventricular hypertrophy,* and your doctor may find it by looking at an electrocardiogram (EKG).

The increased thickness affects the heart's expansion and contraction, which explains why you may be out of breath when you climb a flight of stairs: You're expending energy, and your body needs more oxygen than you're able to distribute. Your heart is not able to pump fast enough to get the oxygen that you need to all parts of your body, and you become winded.

Congestive heart failure and angina also can be results of excess weight. Severe obesity may predispose you to an irregular heartbeat as well as coronary artery disease.

Diabetes

There are two types of diabetes: Type 1 and Type 2. Type 1 diabetes is usually diagnosed in children and adolescents and was previously known as *juvenile diabetes.* Type 2 diabetes, which normally develops in adulthood, is associated with obesity; approximately 80 percent of patients with Type 2 diabetes are overweight. Weight loss is the best treatment for Type 2, or *insulin-resistant,* diabetes. Weight loss and weight loss surgery have resulted in up to 90 percent improvement or resolution of Type 2 diabetes.

Medical treatments do not halt the progression of this disease. Diabetes occurs when either the body is not producing enough insulin or the body is resisting absorbing it. Without insulin, the body is unable to use sugar or glucose to fuel the cells. With high levels of glucose in your blood, damage occurs to your eyes, heart, kidneys, or nerves.

Sleep apnea

Severely obese people commonly have two situations that hinder their breathing when they lie down to sleep. Because severely obese people have a large abdomen, they may notice a shortness of breath as the abdomen interferes with the function of the diaphragm.

A second problem, *sleep apnea,* results when gravity exerts pressure on the thickened tissues and muscles of the throat and neck when lying down. This pressure causes a restriction that blocks the flow of air to the lungs, interrupting the breathing process. A reduction of air reduces the amount of available oxygen to the lungs. In some patients, this condition can affect the rhythm of the heart.

Some severely obese people have a related disease known as *obesity hypoventilation disorder* (OHS). People who suffer from OHS have problems with normal breathing, because the belly pushes up on the diaphragm and the chest wall is heavy and difficult to lift. As this condition progresses, they develop a buildup of carbon dioxide in their bloodstream. The end stage of OHS is also known as Pickwickian syndrome; patients with Pickwickian syndrome have heart failure.

Severely obese patients are frequently short of breath because they aren't able to keep up with the amount of oxygen they need when they're exerting themselves.

Acid reflux

Acid reflux occurs when stomach acid sloshes up through the valve at the top of the stomach into the esophagus, causing heartburn. In more serious cases of acid reflux, stomach acid can eat away the tissue of the esophagus, which can lead to cancer of the esophagus. Many obese people suffer from acid-reflux disease because the belly contents push up on the stomach and back the contents of the stomach into the esophagus.

Osteoarthritis

Osteoarthritis is a common joint disease that affects the knees, hips, and lower back. As your weight increases, excessive pressure is put on these joints, causing the cartilage that cushions the joints to wear away much faster than it does in a person who is not obese.

Polycystic ovary syndrome

Polycystic ovary syndrome (PCOS) is common in as many as 10 percent of women of childbearing years. The syndrome is characterized by the inability of a woman to ovulate or to ovulate infrequently. It also is accompanied by the condition of insulin resistance, which causes the ovaries to increase the production of *androgens* (male hormones). Increased male hormones affect ovulation, so patients have infertility associated with PCOS.

Freeing yourself of serious health problems

Prior to my weight loss surgery, I was becoming diabetic, and my heart wasn't getting enough oxygen. I had a hiatal hernia, gastric reflux, and even water gave me heartburn. I retained so much fluid that it was difficult to bend my knees and I hadn't seen my shins in years. I had such severe lower-back pain that just walking to the mailbox brought tears to my eyes because of the pain from heel spurs. If I did make the trek to the mailbox, I came back out of breath, with my heart pounding.

After my bypass, all that disappeared. After going from a size 24 to a 14/12, I don't have a single health complaint. I no longer have to take any medications, and I'm able to work out five days a week.

Marjorie Schuyler
Greensburg, Pennsylvania

Insulin resistance also can result in weight gain. Many women with PCOS and severe obesity have turned to weight loss surgery to help them with their weight loss, and because the weight loss helps insulin resistance, this seems to jump-start ovulation. Many women with PCOS who have had weight loss surgery have gone on to have healthy pregnancies.

Knowing What You're Getting Into

Weight loss surgery is a life-altering process, and you need to know everything you'll be getting into if you go through with it. Knowledge equals safety and success.

Information can come from a variety of places. Some of the information you find will definitely help you in your journey; other information may be based on rumor or just plain inaccurate. So, consider the source.

In addition to this book, here are some good sources of information on weight loss surgery:

- ✔ **Your surgeon:** Your surgeon most likely will have an informational meeting, usually with a group of people who are new to the idea of weight loss surgery, just as you are. The meetings may be held once or twice a month. Typically, the surgeon will make a presentation, and other members of the surgeon's practice — such as a nurse practitioner or *bariatric coordinator* (normally a nurse who has had special training in bariatrics) — will be there for you to meet. You may watch a video and be given printed information about the surgery and the practice. You'll probably be given forms to complete, in which you'll detail your medical history and your attempts at dieting. You'll also have an opportunity to ask questions.

Take someone with you to the informational meeting, preferably someone who will act as your support following surgery. Having an extra pair of ears is a good idea, in case you miss something. Also, if this is someone who is concerned about your having the surgery, the meeting will give him an opportunity to ask the questions that are on his mind.

✔ **Support groups:** Most medical practices have a support-group meeting once a month. These support groups are excellent sources of information. You'll be able to speak with people who are patients of the practice you're planning to work with. Ask them about their experiences, both good and bad.

✔ **Journals or magazines:** The following journals or magazines all have featured excellent articles on weight loss surgery:

- *Journal of the American Medical Association* (http://jama.ama-assn.org)

- *The New England Journal of Medicine* (www.nejm.org)

- *Obesity Surgery* (www.springer.com/medicine/surgery/journal/11695)

- *Surgery for Obesity and Related Diseases* (www.soard.org)

- *Surgical Endoscopy* (www.springer.com/medicine/surgery/journal/464)

- *Your Weight Matters* (www.obesityaction.org/educational-resources/your-weight-matters-magazine)

✔ **The Internet:** Here are some reputable places where you can get information online:

- **American Society for Metabolic & Bariatric Surgery (**www.asmbs.org**):** The American Society for Metabolic & Bariatric Surgery is a professional organization for surgeons and healthcare professionals and a great source of information for the public.

- **NoObesity.com (**www.noobesity.com**):** This is the website of author and surgeon Marina Kurian, M.D. Here you can find information on the different weight loss procedures, the weight loss program of Dr. Kurian, as well as frequently asked questions.

- **Obesity Action Coalition (**www.obesityaction.org**):** This is a nonprofit organization formed in 2005 to advocate for those affected by obesity and to help obesity education around the country.

- **Obesity Help (**www.obesityhelp.com**):** This site is designed to provide a link to people exploring weight loss surgery. Here you can find peers and surgeons in your area, find out about their experiences, and read comments from patients about surgeons.

- **Obesity Society (**www.obesity.org**):** The Obesity Society is an organization for advocacy and education on obesity.

- **Weight Loss Surgery Center (**www.wlscenter.com**):** This is the website of author Barbara Thompson. Here you can find information presented from a patient's point of view, written by someone who has experienced weight loss surgery and lived and lost weight with it. The website includes success stories, research articles, books, CDs, recipes, and other resources of interest to patients. You also can find links to Barbara's blog and Facebook page, WLS Private. (The Facebook page is private so that others outside the group can't view posts, but interested people can join.)

Here are some sources of *misinformation* on weight loss surgery — well meaning or not:

- ✔ **Friends or relatives:** People who tell you that they know of a friend or relative who had surgery years ago and had complications are not reliable sources of information. Although your family and friends mean well and are concerned for your welfare, they're probably not taking into account the evolution of the field of medicine. Surgery that was done many years ago is not the same as surgery performed today. And you are not identical to the other person they know who had weight loss surgery.

- ✔ **Popular media accounts:** The press has not been kind to the field of weight loss surgery. Sensational and tragic stories are reported excessively. Unfortunately, good news is not what sells. Media reports seldom have sufficient background to use as a source of information. However, they *can* raise a red flag concerning the performance of a certain surgeon or hospital. You can use a media account as a springboard to get more information.

- ✔ **Internet:** The Internet is both a good source of information and a bad source of information, because it's full of — you guessed it — good and bad information. Unhelpful Internet sources include personal accounts and some chat rooms. Chat rooms are great places for support, but they aren't great sources of information. Like popular media accounts, they can alert you to potential problem areas. If a personal website or chat room has raised some questions in your mind, use that as a basis to check out more-reputable sources.

Making a Lifelong Commitment: Are You Ready?

Despite what many people think, weight loss surgery is not the easy way out. Many people mistakenly believe that having weight loss surgery produces instant success. Unfortunately, as an obese person, you're subjected to prejudice because society assumes you could lose weight if only you tried hard enough. People often say, "I lost my weight the old-fashioned way." Well, for people who've struggled with severe weight problems for years and who are severely obese, the old-fashioned way only means struggling to lose weight and then rapidly regaining it. In fact, studies show that people who lose substantial amounts of weight have certain elevations in hormones that can result in weight regain.

Weight loss surgery brings along with it a whole new set of rules to consider before taking that all-important first step. There are no guarantees of success. You need to prepare for changes in other aspects of your life, including your family, career, social life, and ego. You need to consider the following *lifelong* commitments:

- ✔ Taking nutritional supplements
- ✔ Eating small meals that are high in protein
- ✔ Decreasing processed carbohydrates
- ✔ Exercising
- ✔ Committing to regular follow-ups with your surgeon and/or dietitian
- ✔ Severely limiting your consumption of sweets
- ✔ Possibly losing friends who remain overweight and are uncomfortable with your weight loss

Weight loss surgery is not a surgery that is typically undone, so be sure you're committed to a healthier lifestyle *before* making your decision. You want to look better and feel better, but you have to commit to following a new lifestyle in order to reap those rewards.

Some people approach weight loss surgery thinking they'll never have to diet or be careful about their weight again, but that isn't the case. You'll still be the product of the calories you take in and the calories you burn, so calorie counting will always be an important issue. Your weight loss surgery simply gives you a tool to help you control your eating. It's a very powerful tool, but one that you have to use in the right way.

Weight loss surgery for children

Obesity among children is growing at an alarming rate. Some parents are considering surgery for their children, especially as they see severe health problems develop. You want the best for your kids, and your heart breaks when you see them suffering from the effects of obesity — including health problems, relentless teasing from their peers, and difficulty participating in the kinds of activities kids are meant to do (running, playing, jumping, leaping, pretending they're superheroes — your basic kid stuff). Because you've heard and read so much about how obesity may be inherited, you may even feel responsible for how your children are suffering.

The most common form of weight loss surgery results in *malabsorption,* which means that not all the nutrients that patients eat are absorbed. Children who undergo weight loss surgery have to be fully grown so that the malabsorption doesn't affect them developmentally. Some physicians question whether children have the maturity to commit to the lifelong changes that are required in order for the surgery to be a success.

The American Society for Metabolic & Bariatric Surgery has published some guidelines for children and weight loss surgery. Children must have

- A BMI of 35 or above, along with severe health problems such as diabetes or sleep apnea

- A BMI of 40 or above, with less-severe health problems

- A pattern of failed supervised diets over at least a six-month time period

- Reached full height and sexual maturity

- The desire to undergo the surgery (independent of what their parents want)

- Parents who are motivated to help the child follow diet guidelines and exercise following surgery

- An evaluation by a team of medical professionals, including a pediatrician, a psychologist, a dietitian, and a surgeon who has performed several hundred of these procedures on adults

The number of children who have had weight loss surgery is relatively small — so doctors can't know with any certainty whether children who have the surgery face any long-term ill effects. If you're considering weight loss surgery for your child, you won't be able to anticipate the health of your child in the future. Putting your child through weight loss surgery is not a decision to be made lightly.

Talk to your pediatrician and school nurse about local resources that may help your child get his or her weight under control short of surgery. Here are some things to think about:

- The entire family must be willing to make changes in eating.

- The entire family must commit to regular physical activity and changes regarding sedentary activities such as TV watching and computer use.

- The child must be committed to a weight loss program.

- The child's progress must be monitored by someone other than the family, such as a family doctor or dietitian.

- The child must receive positive reinforcement.

- The treatment program must involve small gradual steps.

Helping your child overcome obesity is a gift that will last a lifetime. If one approach doesn't work, try another until you find something that does — and never give up. Your child will thank you for it down the road.

Chapter 3

Incision Decisions: Your Surgical Options

•••

In This Chapter

▶ Understanding that all weight loss surgeries are not alike

▶ Identifying the various types of surgeries and how they work

▶ Recognizing the pros and cons of the most commonly performed surgeries

▶ Familiarizing yourself with lesser-known surgeries

•••

Several types of weight loss surgery exist, and each one differs in how it functions, how it helps you lose weight, and how much weight loss it will likely produce. In this chapter, we cover each type of weight loss surgery — including some of the variations on the routine — and the pros and cons of each.

If you have a choice of surgeries, the information in this chapter will help you decide which one is best for you. If your surgeon has told you which way you should go, this chapter will give you a sense of what your surgery will involve. Most bariatric surgeons specialize in more than one kind of weight loss surgery and can discuss with you the merits of the various procedures. By understanding each of the weight loss surgeries ahead of time, you'll have the basics down and can ask more-specific questions. You also can have a surgery in mind and seek out a surgeon based upon your research.

Roux-en-Y

Roux-en-Y (pronounced roo-en-why, and often abbreviated to RNY) gastric bypass surgery is known as the gold standard of weight loss surgeries. Approximately 60 percent to 70 percent of all surgeries performed in the United States currently are Roux-en-Y.

Digestion 101

Normal digestion begins in the mouth where food is chewed and mixed with saliva. The food then goes down the esophagus and into the stomach, where further digestion takes place as food is mixed with gastric acid. The food stays in the stomach with the help of the pyloric valve. It then enters the three parts of the small intestine —the duodenum, the jejunum, and the ileum where it is mixed with bile and other enzymes, and the food is digested. Absorption of nutrients takes place in the small intestine. Waste then enters the colon and is eventually eliminated.

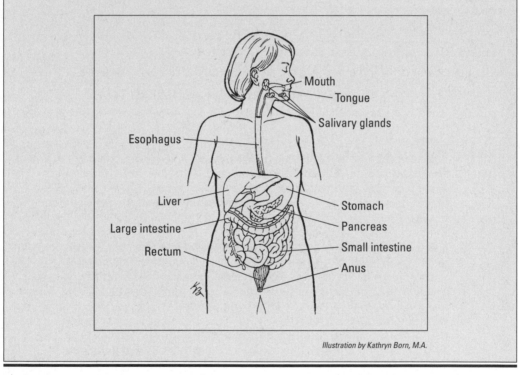

Illustration by Kathryn Born, M.A.

In the 1980s, the term *stomach stapling* referred to the weight loss procedure known as vertical banded gastroplasty (VBG). Unfortunately, some people use the term *stomach stapling* for gastric bypass as well, which is an entirely different procedure. The failure rate with VBG was very high, so when people associate gastric bypass surgery with VBG by calling them both stomach stapling, patients sometimes have the impression that gastric bypass has a high failure rate as well — which is not the case.

What is it?

A Roux-en-Y gastric bypass makes the stomach smaller and bypasses some of the small intestine. The stomach is made smaller by dividing the stomach with staples into two compartments or by partitioning the stomach with staples. Today, surgeons commonly divide the stomach while partitioning it. In the laparoscopic procedure, the stomach must be divided. The smaller stomach is referred to as the *pouch.* The size of the pouch is about 1 to 2 ounces, or roughly the size of an egg. (As a contrast, the size of a normal stomach is about the size of a football.)

The small intestine is divided at a certain length by using a stapler. Of the two cut ends of small intestine, the intestine that was farther away is brought up to the new stomach pouch, and this new hookup is called a *gastrojejunostomy.* Some people also refer to this as the *proximal anastomosis.* The other cut end of small intestine is then plugged back into the intestine to complete the circuit, and this new attachment is called the *distal anastomosis.* The small intestine that is attached to the stomach is known as the *Roux limb.* The other cut end of small intestine is known as the *biliopancreatic limb,* because it contains the bile from the liver and the enzymes to digest food from the pancreas. When the biliopancreatic limb joins the Roux limb, the small intestine is known as the *common channel,* and this is where the majority of the food is digested and calories are absorbed. Figure 3-1 illustrates the Roux-en-Y gastric bypass procedure.

When you have Roux-en-Y surgery, after you chew food and it mixes with saliva in your mouth, the food goes down the esophagus into the new stomach pouch and then into the small intestine. The bile and other enzymes don't join the food until further down the intestine, so there is less time for food digestion and calorie absorption.

Who does it work for?

If you need help with portion control, you may be a good candidate for a Roux-en-Y. The small pouch will keep you from overeating. When you eat more than your pouch holds, you'll feel a pain or discomfort in your chest and will likely throw up the food.

If you have trouble controlling sweets, you also may be a good candidate, because of dumping syndrome. (See Chapter 18 for more information.)

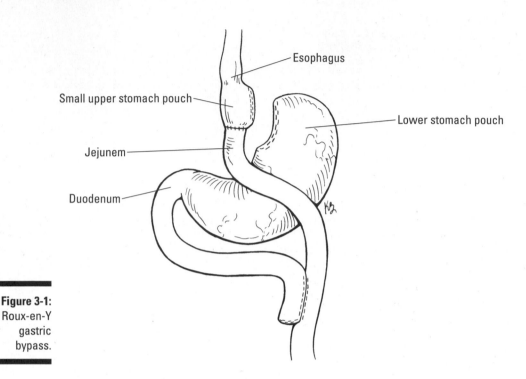

Esophagus

Small upper stomach pouch

Lower stomach pouch

Jejunem

Duodenum

Figure 3-1:
Roux-en-Y
gastric
bypass.

Illustration by Kathryn Born, M.A.

What are the pros and cons?

Here are the advantages that the Roux-en-Y gastric bypass surgery offers to patients:

- ✔ Up to 96 percent of patients see a remission of or improvement in their diabetes.

- ✔ Up to 90 percent of patients see a remission of or improvement in their high blood pressure.

- ✔ Up to 80 percent of patients see a remission of or improvement in their sleep apnea.

- ✔ Patients see a lessening of pain related to osteoarthritis.

- ✔ Patients see a lessening of their gastroesophageal reflux disease (GERD) symptoms.

- ✔ Some patients see an improvement in their fertility.

- ✔ Patients experience great weight loss. Patients can maintain an average of 65 percent to 70 percent of excess weight loss at five years after surgery. In other words, they can expect to lose 65 percent to 70 percent of the amount that they're overweight.

✔ Patients experience better long-term weight loss than with diet, exercise, and medication.

✔ On average, patients experience more weight loss than with behavioral modification.

✔ Patients are less likely to gain back the weight they've lost than are patients of some of the other weight loss procedures.

✔ Patients experience rapid weight loss, and they can achieve most of the weight loss within the first year.

✔ The small gastric pouch forces patients to modify their diets.

✔ Some patients experience dumping syndrome if they eat something too high in sugar or fat (see Chapter 18 for more information), which keeps them away from high-sugar or high-fat foods.

Though it's the most popular form of weight loss surgery performed today, Roux-en-Y does have drawbacks:

✔ Because the stomach is divided and the small intestine is rerouted, leakages can occur right after surgery.

✔ Because Roux-en-Y is surgery, it can involve complications such as *pulmonary embolism* (a blood clot in the lungs), bleeding, infection, *stricture* (a severe narrowing of the hookup of the stomach to the intestine due to scar tissue), hernia, and even death.

✔ Ulcers can occur at the hookup of the stomach to the intestine.

✔ You may regain some of the weight you've lost if you don't watch your diet and follow an exercise regimen.

✔ You may have gas, and it could smell worse than it did before surgery (though your doctor can help with this).

✔ For the rest of your life, you're at a slight risk for intestinal obstruction.

✔ You have to modify your diet.

✔ You may experience more frequent bowel movements or constipation.

✔ You may experience nutritional deficiencies, which means you'll have to take nutritional supplements for the rest of your life.

✔ You may experience dumping syndrome if you eat something too high in sugar or fat (see Chapter 18); although this can motivate you to avoid high-sugar or high-fat foods, dumping syndrome is no fun.

✔ The surgery to reverse Roux-en-Y gastric bypass is more difficult than Roux-en-Y itself, so it's only reversed in extreme situations.

After your gastric bypass, call your surgeon if you experience any abdominal problems or any other new concerns. He may have seen a similar problem in other patients.

How much is bypassed?

Gastric bypass surgeries are classified by the amount of small intestine that is bypassed. Or put another way, the length of the Roux limb. In a proximal gastric bypass, 150 cm or less are bypassed. In a distal gastric bypass, more than 150 cm are bypassed. A longer Roux limb may increase the amount of weight loss in the super-severely obese.

Adjustable Gastric Banding

Adjustable gastric banding is the simplest of all the weight loss procedures. The surgery is less invasive than the Roux-en-Y gastric bypass or the duodenal switch surgeries.

What is it?

An adjustable band is placed around the upper stomach and sewn in place (see Figure 3-2). A balloon on the inside of the band sits against the stomach. The band has tubing that is connected to a port that is inserted under the skin and secured to the abdominal wall muscle. This port can be accessed with a special needle. The balloon is blown up or adjusted by putting saline through a needle into the port. The saline travels through the body by way of the tubing and then into the balloon. When the balloon is inflated, the band tightens around the stomach, essentially slowing down the passage of food through the band. This gives you the sense that your stomach is full, and if you eat another bite, you may throw up. Because your intestinal anatomy is not altered, every calorie you eat is absorbed. There is no problem with malabsorption the way there is with the Roux-en-Y gastric bypass. Sometimes, a hiatal hernia is repaired when the band is placed around the stomach to decrease the chance of heartburn or reflux.

Who does it work for?

You may be a good candidate for adjustable gastric banding if you're well disciplined and willing to go through a slower weight loss than what a Roux-en-Y gastric bypass patient experiences. Because the weight loss tends to be less than it is in Roux-en-Y gastric bypass surgery, patients with gastric banding have to work harder in order to achieve similar weight loss. Because patients don't experience the dumping syndrome that they can with gastric bypass, adjustable gastric banding patients can sabotage the surgery by drinking high-calorie liquids such as milkshakes.

If you undergo adjustable gastric banding, you must be committed to having the balloon on the band inflated, which adjusts the restriction. These adjustments are called *fills*. Fills are performed for hunger, portion size, and weight loss. Band patients are seen more often in the first year than patients who've had other weight loss procedures.

The Lap-Band (made by Allergan) and the Realize Band (made by Johnson & Johnson) are the two bands approved by the U.S. Food and Drug Administration (FDA). At least three other adjustable bands are available in Europe. Both the Lap-Band and the Realize Band are adjustable and work by making you eat less food.

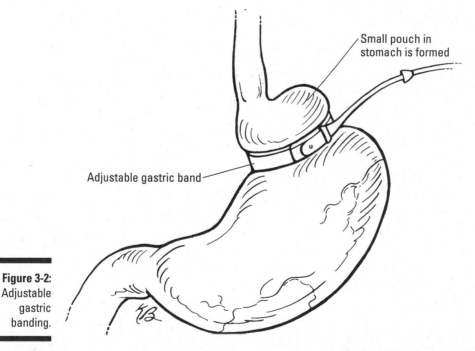

Small pouch in stomach is formed

Adjustable gastric band

Figure 3-2: Adjustable gastric banding.

Illustration by Kathryn Born, M.A.

Variations on the Roux-en-Y

Your surgeon may decide to perform one of several slight variations on the Roux-en-Y procedure, such as the following:

✔ **Fobi pouch (see the following figure):** The Fobi pouch is a gastric bypass with a variation. Dr. Mal Fobi designed this operation to try to prevent late weight regain. The premise is that a band around the pouch above the new hookup of the stomach to the intestine will continue to give patients long-term restriction, because the band acts as a gate to allow food to pass slowly into the intestine. The band can be made of silicone or Marlex, depending on the surgeon's preference.

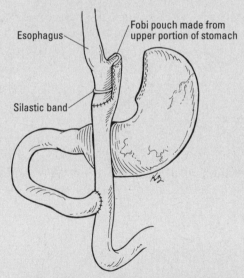

Esophagus

Fobi pouch made from upper portion of stomach

Silastic band

Illustration by Kathryn Born, M.A.

✔ **Adjustable gastric band and bypass:** Some surgeons place an adjustable gastric band around the stomach pouch so that the restriction can be adjusted. This procedure is done today for gastric bypass patients who have regained much of the weight they originally lost.

✔ **Mini gastric bypass (see the following figure):** The mini gastric bypass is not a new procedure, but it is a new procedure for weight loss. This procedure, like the gastric bypass, was originally done for stomach ulcers. A long, thin stomach pouch is created with staples. A loop of small intestine is then brought up to the new pouch. The small intestine is not divided, so there is only one new hookup. This procedure may result in a high rate of ulcers around the hookup. A few studies have been conducted comparing the Roux-en-Y gastric bypass to the mini gastric bypass, and the data show that the weight loss is approximately the same. This operation has been carefully evaluated by the American Society for Metabolic & Bariatric Surgery (ASMBS), which has found that there is little role for this operation in present-day weight loss surgery.

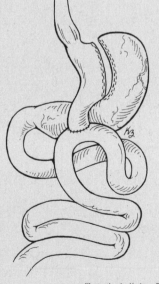

Illustration by Kathryn Born, M.A.

What are the pros and cons?

Adjustable gastric banding has some definite advantages, including the following:

- The intestine is not rerouted or cut.

- Patients are in control of their weight loss because they control how tight or loose the band is by going to their surgeon for fills.

- Some patients see up to 85 percent remission of or improvement in their diabetes.

- Patients see up to 70 percent remission of or improvement in their high blood pressure.

- Patients see a lessening of pain related to osteoarthritis.

- Patients see a lessening of GERD symptoms.

- Some patients see an improvement in fertility.

- Patients experience great weight loss and can maintain an average of 55 percent of excess weight loss five years after surgery. In other words, they can expect to lose 55 percent of the amount that they're overweight.

- On average, patients experience greater weight loss than with diet, exercise, and medication.

- On average, patients experience greater weight loss than with behavioral modification.

- Patients don't have to take nutritional supplements.

- The band can be removed easily if necessary, so the surgery is reversible.

- It's the least expensive weight loss procedure to perform, which may be a consideration if you need to pay for your procedure yourself.

- Patients don't experience dumping syndrome.

As with any procedure, adjustable gastric banding does have some cons, including the following:

- It is surgery and, as with any surgery, you may experience complications, including leakage, pulmonary embolism, bleeding, infection, hernia, and even death.

- Because you're in control, you may regain some of the weight you lose if you don't watch your diet and follow an exercise regimen.

- You may experience bloating, burping, or flatulence.

- You may have left shoulder pain, which is due to gas trapped in your upper stomach.

✔ You may experience problems with the band that may require more surgery. For example, you may experience port problems, tubing problems, *band erosion* (where the band actually makes a hole in the stomach), and *gastric prolapse* (where the stomach below the band slips up through the band).

✔ You may experience heartburn or GERD symptoms that require significant loosening of your band.

✔ You may need to have the band removed because you have trouble tolerating it, either for physical or psychological reasons.

✔ Patients do not experience dumping syndrome (considered as a con by some patients and surgeons, because dumping helps patients to avoid sweets).

✔ If the banding is adjusted too tight, you may eat foods that are either really soft or really crunchy so the food can pass through the band without making you feel like it's stuck. Usually, these types of foods are extremely high in calories (like a milkshake), so you may end up gaining weight. This type of maladaptive eating also can occur with gastric bypass, but it's less likely with gastric bypass than it is with adjustable gastric banding.

Sleeve Gastrectomy

The sleeve gastrectomy was originally part of a more complex operation, the biliopancreatic diversion with duodenal switch. Surgeons started to do just part of this operation, removing part of the stomach, in patients who were too sick to undergo a more extensive procedure.

What is it?

Sleeve gastrectomy (shown in Figure 3-3) involves removing the outer curve of the stomach and creating a stomach that holds about ½ cup of food. The *pylorus,* which regulates the entry of food into the intestine, is not removed, and food enters the intestine normally. The operation gave high-risk patients substantial weight loss, so surgeons started performing it as a standalone weight loss procedure.

The part of the stomach that is removed also makes a hormone that makes you hungry. When this part of the stomach is gone, you won't be as hungry as you were before the surgery.

Who does it work for?

If you need help with portion control, you may be a good candidate for a sleeve gastrectomy. The smaller stomach will keep you from overeating. When you eat more than your stomach holds, you'll feel a pain or discomfort in your chest and will likely throw up the food.

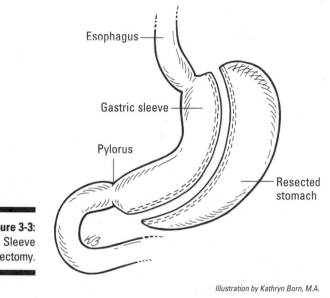

Esophagus

Gastric sleeve

Pylorus

Resected stomach

Figure 3-3: Sleeve gastrectomy.

Illustration by Kathryn Born, M.A.

TECHNICAL STUFF

On the cutting edge: The NOTES technique

With the goal of causing less tissue damage and performing surgery without scars, surgeons began to think about going down through the mouth or sometimes up through the vagina to perform certain abdominal procedures like removing the gallbladder, appendix, or spleen. This technique is called natural orifice transluminal endoscopic surgery (NOTES), and it has been used to perform sleeve gastrectomies.

There is some controversy regarding opening another organ to do a procedure just to prevent a scar on the abdominal wall. Surgeon advocates of NOTES feel that there is less pain associated with the technique. As of this writing, however, the risks and benefits have not been clearly identified. NOTES is considered an investigational technique, and the surgeons doing it send all their data to a registry so the proposed benefits and risks can be tracked.

What are the pros and cons?

Here are the advantages that sleeve gastrectomy surgery offers to patients:

- ✔ Up to 85 percent of patients see a remission of or improvement in their diabetes.

- ✔ Up to 75 percent of patients see a remission of or improvement in their high blood pressure.

- ✔ Up to 70 percent of patients see a remission of or improvement in their sleep apnea.

- ✔ Patients see a lessening of pain related to osteoarthritis.

- ✔ Some patients see an improvement in their fertility.

- ✔ Patients experience great weight loss. Patients can maintain an average of 55 percent to 60 percent of excess weight loss at five years after surgery. In other words, they can expect to lose 55 percent to 60 percent of the amount that they're overweight.

- ✔ Patients experience better long-term weight loss than with diet, exercise, and medication.

- ✔ On average, patients experience more weight loss than with behavioral modification.

- ✔ Patients are less likely to gain back the weight they've lost because they aren't as hungry.

- ✔ Patients experience rapid weight loss, and they can achieve most of the weight loss within the first year.

- ✔ The smaller stomach forces patients to modify their diets.

Though it's gaining popularity as a weight loss procedure today, sleeve gastrectomy does have some drawbacks:

- ✔ Because the stomach is removed and there is a long staple line, leakages can occur right after surgery.

- ✔ If a leak occurs, you may need other procedures or reoperations to try to heal the leak.

- ✔ As with any abdominal surgery, it can involve complications such as pulmonary embolism, bleeding, infection, stricture, hernia, and even death.

- ✔ Part of the remaining stomach can narrow as it heals, causing a stricture that may need to be dilated or stretched out with a balloon.

- ✔ You may regain some of the weight you've lost if you don't watch your diet and follow an exercise regimen.

- ✔ You have to modify your diet.

- ✔ Because part of the stomach is removed, the surgery is not reversible.

Biliopancreatic Diversion

The biliopancreatic diversion is a procedure in which part of the stomach is actually removed and an intestinal bypass is performed. The biliopancreatic diversion can be performed in two ways, and the difference between the two procedures lies in which part of the stomach is removed.

What is it?

In the biliopancreatic diversion (see Figure 3-4), the lower part of the stomach is removed, and the remaining stomach is hooked up to the part of the small intestine that is closer to the colon, known as the *ileum*. In the biliopancreatic diversion with duodenal switch (see Figure 3-5), the outer curve of the stomach is removed, and the first part of the small intestine is hooked up to the ileum.

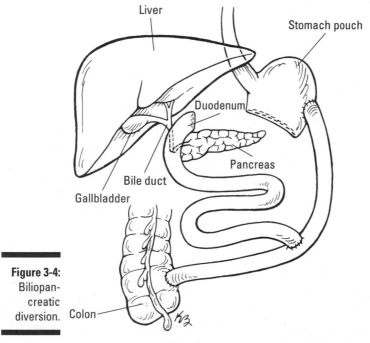

Figure 3-4:
Biliopancreatic diversion.

Illustration by Kathryn Born, M.A.

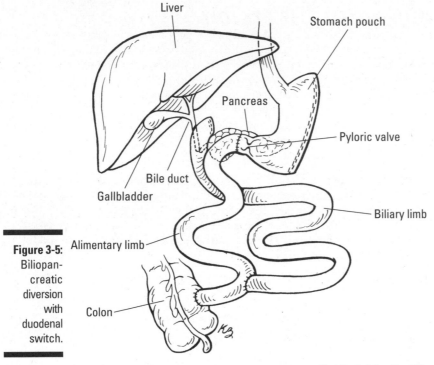

Figure 3-5:
Biliopan-
creatic
diversion
with
duodenal
switch.

Illustration by Kathryn Born, M.A.

Approximately 90 percent of the small intestine is bypassed in both the surgeries, resulting in significantly fewer calories and nutrients being absorbed. The stomach that remains holds approximately ½ cup to 1 cup.

The dumping syndrome that can occur with gastric bypass doesn't usually occur with the biliopancreatic diversion. This weight loss procedure has the least likelihood of weight regain, but it also has the highest complication rate.

Who does it work for?

You may be a good candidate for the biliopancreatic diversion if you have a great deal of weight to lose. It also may be a good option for you if you don't think you can eat very small quantities for the rest of your life and if you'll be especially diligent about taking supplements and eating enough protein. Because 90 percent of the intestine is bypassed, you have to eat more-than-normal amounts of protein to get your body what it needs. You have to commit to the follow-up, meaning that you have to see your surgeon or your primary-care doctor because of the risk of nutritional problems. Blood work should be checked every six months for the rest of your life.

Laparoscopic versus open procedures

In an *open* procedure, a single long cut is used to gain access to the abdomen. The surgeon uses his eyes to see the contents of the abdomen and his hands to perform surgery.

In a *laparoscopic* procedure, many small incisions less than 1 inch in length are used to access the abdomen. Through these small incisions, a long, thin tube (a *laparoscope*) attached to a camera is inserted into the abdomen, and the abdomen is viewed on a television screen in the operating room. Different long, thin instruments are used to move the organs around and perform the surgery. Usually for laparoscopic weight loss surgery, five to six small incisions are used.

However, one of the newer techniques in surgery is a single-incision technique for laparoscopic procedures, including gastric banding and sleeve gastrectomy. Generally, one incision is made at the belly button to try to hide the scar. The procedure itself is still done with laparoscopic instruments. The only benefit to this type of approach in surgery is cosmetic. Many studies don't show a difference in pain level or recovery between traditional laparoscopy and the single-incision laparoscopic technique. On the downside, because there is a bigger incision at the belly button, there is a small possibility of developing a belly button hernia down the line.

Laparoscopy also can be performed robotically. In robotic surgery, your surgeon is still performing the procedure laparoscopically, but she's sitting at a console in the operating room and controlling the laparoscopic instruments from there. Some surgeons prefer to use robotic technology; other surgeons prefer standard laparoscopy. There is no benefit to the robotic technique — it's just a matter of which technique your surgeon prefers.

So, how do you choose between laparoscopic surgery and open surgery? Here are the advantages of laparoscopic surgery:

✔ The surgeon can visualize the abdomen better. The abdominal organs are magnified and the laparoscope can reveal some hard-to-see areas of the abdomen.

✔ Smaller incisions mean fewer wound complications (lower risk of infection and hernias, for example).

✔ Patients experience less pain after surgery.

✔ Patients get moving sooner after surgery.

✔ Patients don't have to stay in the hospital as long.

The advantages of open surgery include the following:

✔ Some surgeons like to hold the organs in their hands.

✔ Some surgeons think they're able to see better.

✔ Some surgeons have more experience with this technique.

The bottom line: If you're comfortable with your surgeon's track record with weight loss surgery, the approach she uses is appropriate. In other words, if your surgeon does great weight loss surgery and happens to do it open rather than laparoscopically, that's okay. If your surgeon does great weight loss surgery and does it laparoscopically, that's okay, too. The surgery performed will be the same surgery whether it's done open or laparoscopically. The only thing that's different is how the surgeon accesses your internal organs.

Note: In some cases, if a surgeon starts with the laparoscopic approach, he may have to make a big incision to complete the operation. This can occur because of significant scar tissue from previous surgeries, bleeding, or difficulty with a particular part of a procedure.

What are the pros and cons?

Here are the advantages of the biliopancreatic diversion (with or without duodenal switch):

✔ Up to 96 percent of patients see a remission of or improvement in their diabetes.

✔ Up to 90 percent of patients see a remission of or improvement in their high blood pressure.

✔ Up to 80 percent of patients see a remission of or improvement in their sleep apnea.

✔ Patients see a lessening in their pain related to osteoarthritis.

✔ Patients see a lessening in their GERD symptoms.

✔ Some patients see an improvement in fertility.

✔ Patients experience significant weight loss. Patients can maintain an average of 75 percent to 80 percent of excess weight loss ten years after surgery. In other words, they can expect to lose 75 percent to 80 percent of the amount that they're overweight.

✔ On average, patients experience greater weight loss than with diet, exercise, and medication.

✔ On average, patients experience greater weight loss than with behavioral modification.

✔ Patients are less likely to gain the weight they've lost than are patients of some of the other weight loss procedures.

As with any procedure, the biliopancreatic diversion (with or without duodenal switch) has some negatives:

✔ Part of the stomach is removed, and the small intestine is divided and rerouted, so leakages can occur.

✔ Because this is surgery, complications — such as pulmonary embolism, bleeding, *pancreatitis* (an inflammation if the pancreas), infection, stricture, hernia, and even death — may occur.

✔ Patients are at risk for liver failure.

✔ Ulcers can occur at the hookup of the stomach to the intestine.

✔ Patients often experience very smelly gas.

✔ You may have four to eight bowel movements per day, depending on what you eat.

✔ For the rest of your life, you're at a slight risk for intestinal obstruction.

    ✔ The intestinal bypass may result in severe nutritional deficiencies, night blindness, brittle bone disease, and protein malnutrition.

    ✔ You have to take nutritional supplements for the rest of your life.

    ✔ Because a part of the stomach is removed, this surgery is not reversible.

Other Weight Loss Procedures

In the following sections, we give you some information on other weight loss procedures that are either new or rarely performed in the United States today.

Vertical banded gastroplasty

Vertical banded gastroplasty (VBG) was originally performed for weight loss in the 1980s and is still performed today. In this procedure, the stomach is partitioned using staples, so you have a smaller pouch that empties into the rest of the stomach (see Figure 3-6). The outlet of the new pouch where it empties into the new stomach is banded with a strip of synthetic material. This procedure is similar to the gastric banding procedure, but it isn't adjustable. Because the stomach is partitioned using staples, the staples can open up, allowing food to pass from the pouch to the rest of the stomach. When this happens, the restriction is gone, and you can eat normally.

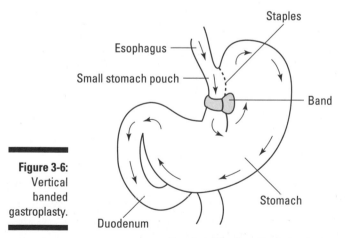

Figure 3-6:
Vertical
banded
gastroplasty.

Illustration by Wiley, Composition Services Graphics

There is a high rate of weight regain with this procedure, so most surgeons do not perform it. Individual surgeons have achieved a higher success rate with this procedure for their patients than the average, but intensive counseling, education, behavior modification, and follow-up are necessary in order to achieve success. Patients may modify their eating behaviors (eating particular soft or crunchy foods to reduce a feeling of tightness in the abdomen), because the restriction is the same from the first day the procedure is done. The band around the outlet of the pouch to the stomach can cause strictures and can erode into the stomach. Both of those situations require corrective surgery.

Nonadjustable gastric banding

Some surgeons place a synthetic band around the upper portion of the stomach that doesn't have a balloon or any method of adjusting it at a later date. This procedure is rarely performed.

Stomach (intragastric) balloons

In this procedure (shown in Figure 3-7), a balloon is placed inside the stomach endoscopically, through the mouth and esophagus. The balloon is then inflated with sterile saline. The procedure works for weight loss, because part of your stomach is filled by the balloon so less food can fit in it. This device is not FDA approved and is used in the United States only under a research protocol.

A stomach balloon is not a long-term solution, because the stomach will expand to accommodate the balloon and more food. However, doctors outside the United States have had reasonable success with intragastric balloons for short-term weight loss in high-risk patients. In other words, the balloon gets some of the weight off people who are too sick to have an abdominal surgery and makes those people better candidates for surgery.

The balloon can deflate by itself and eventually move into the intestines and can get stuck. If this happens, surgery is required to remove the balloon and relieve the blockage.

Endobarriers

The Endobarrier gastrointestinal liner is an endoscopic weight loss method. A long flexible tube is placed from the end of the esophagus, through the stomach, and into the second part of the small intestine to act as a bypass without surgery. Food that's eaten bypasses the stomach and part of the intestine. Not all the calories are absorbed, and beneficial effects on blood sugar have been observed. The Endobarrier has been approved outside the United States to treat obesity and type 2 diabetes, but it is not FDA approved. Therefore, it is considered investigational in the United States and can be placed only under a research protocol at this time.

Gastric greater curve plication

Because making the stomach smaller with the sleeve gastrectomy has been so successful, some surgeons have started to make the stomach smaller by folding it in on itself with sutures. This procedure is performed laparoscopically. Because the stomach is not cut, the risk of leakage is less than with a sleeve gastrectomy. You eat a lot less and lose weight. How much weight you can lose and how long the weight loss lasts have not been well established. As of this writing, relatively few procedures of this type have been performed and mostly outside the United States. The procedure is considered investigational, and the ASMBS recommends performing it under a research protocol.

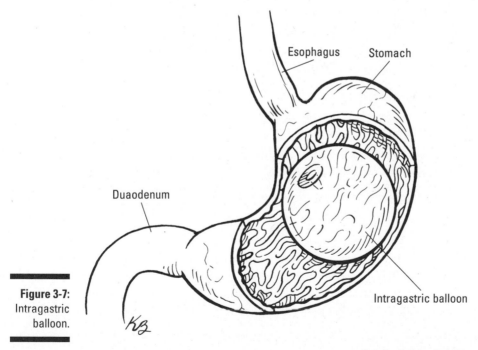

Esophagus   Stomach

Duaodenum

Figure 3-7:
Intragastric
balloon.

Intragastric balloon

Illustration by Kathryn Born, M.A.

Metabolic surgery

If you have diabetes, high blood pressure, high cholesterol or triglycerides and sleep apnea, you have something called *metabolic syndrome,* and it needs to be treated to prevent heart attacks and death. Surgeons operating for severe obesity have always seen improvements in metabolic syndrome and each of these health conditions. But some surgeons started to think of ways to treat not just obesity but metabolic syndrome directly. Metabolic surgery is different from the biliopancreatic diversion with duodenal switch and the Roux-en-Y gastric bypass. Different types of intestinal bypasses with or without a sleeve gastrectomy have been studied to see which operation would have the greatest success in curing type 2 diabetes and treating metabolic syndrome.

In patients who don't qualify for traditional weight loss surgery because of their body mass index (those with a BMI less than 35) but who have these health conditions, metabolic surgery has been used with great success. The greatest improvement has been seen in patients with type 2 diabetes. Metabolic surgery is still considered investigational and is done under a research protocol at this time.

Chapter 4

Understanding the Risks of Surgery

As with any surgery, weight loss surgery brings with it certain risks. Choosing to have weight loss surgery isn't about ignoring those risks — it's about understanding them and deciding whether the rewards are worth the risks.

In this chapter, we identify some of the more common complications that can occur with weight loss surgery. This chapter is by no means a complete list; we don't mention every possible complication here — just the more common ones.

Be sure to talk with your surgeon about the potential complications. If you have more questions about anything you read in this chapter, bring it up with your surgeon and get his or her take on it. Your health situation is unique, because there's no one else exactly like you — your surgeon will know better than anybody what risks and complications you face.

Gastrointestinal Leaks

In the world of weight loss surgery, a leak occurs when something that should have been watertight is not. Sounds a lot like the pipes under your sink, doesn't it?

Unlike your kitchen sink, of course, your surgeon can't just open the cupboard doors and see the pool of water. So, how does your surgeon diagnose a leak? Here are some of the signs she'll look for:

- Your heart rate may be high.
- Your urine output may be low.
- You may complain of worsening abdominal pain.
- You may have a high fever.
- Your white blood cell count may be rising.
- Your kidney function may get worse.
- An upper GI series or abdominal CAT scan may show the leak.

No single sign is absolute. A leak can be very frightening for weight loss surgery patients, but the important thing is discovering it. After a leak is detected, your surgeon can deal with it — the leaks that are not discovered are the ones that are dangerous. Fortunately, leaks occur only in 1 percent to 2 percent of all procedures.

At the end of your operation, your surgeon may leave a drain that comes out of your belly wall. The drain gives your doctor an idea what's going on inside. The drains are made of a very soft and flexible plastic, and they don't hurt. The only downside of these drains is that they can become clogged, so they don't always show what's going on inside your belly (such as a leak or an infection). Your doctor will look for other signs to figure out whether you're having these kinds of problems.

If you have a leak from a gastric bypass, sleeve, or biliopancreatic diversion (with or without duodenal switch) procedure, your doctor may have several options:

- **If a drain is already in place and it's draining the leak and your body functions are tolerating the leak, the doctor can leave the drain in place and give you antibiotics and intravenous nutrition.** If all goes well, your leak will heal on its own.

✔ **If you don't have a drain, you may need to have a drain placed; if your current drain is not working correctly, you may need to have another drain placed.** Placement of a drain can be done either by a special radiologist (called an *interventional radiologist*) or by your surgeon, which requires a trip back to the operating room. If you're taken back to the operating room, your surgeon will try to stop the leak by making the area watertight if possible, and drains will be placed in the area. The most important part of this re-operation is to drain the area that's leaking. Despite this intervention, the area can still leak. You may or may not be fed through your intestines, and you may or may not receive intravenous nutrition to allow your body time and nourishment to try to heal the leak.

✔ **Sometimes your leak may be better treated by using a stent.** A *stent* is a tubular structure that can be placed within the new stomach that can cover the hole or leak. It keeps your saliva and stomach juices inside your GI tract. The stent is placed endoscopically (through the mouth) and can be performed by your surgeon or a gastroenterologist.

Leaks also can occur in gastric-banding procedures. For example, a leak can occur in the stomach or the intestines due to an injury to that organ during the surgery. This is known as a *perforation;* it occurs less than 1 percent of the time. If you have a perforation, you'll likely require another operation to fix the problem.

With gastric banding, an *erosion* (a chronic hole in the stomach that occurs over time) also can occur. This requires further surgery to remove the band and fix the hole. If you have an erosion, you'll still be a candidate for further weight loss surgery. The timing and the type of surgery are some things that are decided between you and your surgeon.

Sometimes, a leak can become a *fistula* (a hole in an organ — usually the stomach in weight loss surgery — that connects to another organ or structure). Fistulas usually form because of a leak in the staple line. This is why fistulas are very unusual in gastric-banding patients — there is no stapling or dividing of tissue. Sometimes fistulas close on their own; other times, surgery or stenting is needed to help close the fistula.

Nutrition is key to help your body heal if you develop a fistula. Your surgeon may ask you not to eat or drink anything by mouth and give you special intravenous nutrition. You may need to have a special surgically placed tube for nutrition, either in a bypassed stomach (if you're a gastric-bypass patient) or in the first part of the small intestine or jejunum.

Sometimes a fistula forms between the stomach pouch and the bypassed stomach in a gastric bypass; in this case, it's known as a *gastrogastric fistula.* A fistula also can connect the stomach to the skin; this is called a *gastrocutaneous fistula.*

Gastric Distention

In gastric bypass surgery, the *remnant* (bypassed stomach) can get distended or blown up and occasionally leak as a result of that distension. This occurs up to 1 percent of the time. If you have gastric distension, you may experience nausea, abdominal pain, hiccups, or sweating. Gastric distension is very difficult to diagnose because the symptoms are so vague. It can be identified by an abdominal X-ray or CAT scan.

If you're experiencing this problem, you'll need a drainage tube placed in the distended stomach. (This procedure can be performed by your surgeon or by an interventional radiologist.) That tube will come out through your skin and drain to a special drainage bag. The tube will stay in place for two to four weeks, sometimes longer. The tube usually is removed in your surgeon's office.

Deep Venous Thrombosis and Pulmonary Embolism

Deep venous thrombosis (DVT) is a potential side effect of weight loss surgery. DVT is a blood clot in one of the deep veins in your leg, arm, neck, or pelvis. It isn't phlebitis, which is a clot and inflammation in a *superficial* vein in your leg, arm, or neck. Clots in the *deep* veins can break off and go to the lungs, which is called *pulmonary embolism.* This is why DVT is such a serious complication.

Blood clots can form during or after any surgery because you're immobile while under anesthesia and, if you don't make the effort to get up and move after surgery, you may be immobile afterward. Some patients come into the hospital for surgery with blood clots already present, because they haven't been very mobile at home.

If you develop a clot in one of your deep veins, you'll probably be put on a blood thinner, which prevents blood clots from forming. The idea is that if your blood can't form clots, the clot you have can't get bigger, which will give your body time to either absorb the clot or bypass the clot.

So, what happens if a blood clot breaks off and goes to your lungs? Your lungs will have a harder time putting oxygen in your blood. To compensate, your heart beats faster and you breathe faster. These attempts to compensate for the pulmonary embolism may not be enough. Usually, you'll need to be put in the hospital on oxygen and a blood thinner. In some cases, the heart and lungs can't compensate for the pulmonary embolism, and you can die.

DVT and pulmonary embolism occur in at least 2 percent to 3 percent of weight loss surgery patients. Death from pulmonary embolism occurs in under 1 percent of weight loss surgery patients.

What can you do to prevent blood clots? Your surgeon will likely have you do one or two of the following:

- ✓ **Take a prophylactic or preventive dose of blood thinner sometime before surgery and continue taking it for some time after the surgery.**

- ✓ **Wear special stockings during the surgery and when you're in the hospital bed after surgery.**

- ✓ **Walk the same day of surgery and during the rest of your recovery.**

- ✓ **Have a special filter placed in the largest vein in your body, which can catch any blood clots that break off from the legs or the pelvic veins.** Not everyone needs a filter. Your doctor will look at your risk profile and decide if you need one.

  Having a filter is not all it's cracked up to be. Yes, it may prevent life-ending blood clots from going to the lungs, but there is a 10 percent rate of complications associated with having the filter stay in your vein long term. A removable filter can be removed up to six months after it's placed, but it can't always be removed.

Bleeding

After weight loss surgery, you can bleed, you can clot, and, unfortunately, you can do both at the same time.

Bleeding can occur with any major surgery. In the case of weight loss surgery, the liver and spleen sit right next to the stomach and can get injured during the surgery. Bleeding from the liver usually stops during the procedure. Bleeding from the spleen may stop, but you may require a *splenectomy* (removal of the spleen).

Either way, you may need a blood transfusion. With gastric bypass, sleeve gastrectomy, and duodenal switch, bleeding can occur from staple lines in addition to the spleen. Your doctor will stop the blood thinner, if you're getting it, and he'll ask you to walk when your blood count stabilizes. While you're in bed, though, flex your ankles and contract your leg and arm muscles as often as possible to prevent blood clots.

Your doctor will have asked you to stop any aspirin or ibuprofen products for a week to ten days before surgery. Aspirin and ibuprofen affect your platelets, which are very important for blood clots to form. This means you can bleed too much when the surgeon is operating. Blood thinners that you get during surgery allow the platelets to form plugs to stop bleeding but affect clot formation in different ways to stop clots from forming in your deep veins. Remember to take only acetaminophen products (for example, Tylenol) before surgery — no ibuprofen (for example, Advil or Motrin) or aspirin. If you're on aspirin and/or Plavix, check with your surgeon to see what you should do. Your surgeon also may want you to stop fish oil, vitamin E, and other herbal supplements, because some of these supplements can make you prone to bleeding.

Some people are more prone to blood clots. This tendency may run in families. Ask your family members if anyone has ever had a blood clot with or without surgery. A *hematologist* (blood specialist) will perform blood tests to see how well your blood clots. If you're prone to blood clots, you'll need to be on life-long medication to keep your blood thin.

How thin is thin enough? With anticoagulants, blood levels can be checked to try to get the blood thinned to an acceptable range. Too little thinning of the blood can result in more blood clots, and too much thinning of the blood can result in bleeding. Bleeding can occur even if your blood levels are in the acceptable range. Long term, the complications of blood clots in the deep veins of the arm or leg can result in persistent swelling of the limb.

Heart Problems

Heart disease is worsened by obesity. In the following sections, we cover some of the heart problems that can occur after weight loss surgery.

Heart attacks

A heart attack can occur after any surgery, and your doctor will try to prevent you from having a heart attack. He'll ask about your personal medical history and your family medical history. If you're considered high risk, as part of your pre-op workup, you'll undergo an EKG and possibly a stress test and/or echocardiogram. You may need a *cardiac catheterization,* which is a dye study of the blood vessels that supply oxygen to your heart.

If you do have a heart attack after the surgery, you'll have an EKG, an echo-cardiogram, and possibly a cardiac catheterization. You'll be moved to a special ward known as the intensive care unit (ICU) or the cardiac care unit (CCU). A cardiologist will follow you, in addition to your surgeon following you, and you'll be given certain special medications to help your heart.

Heart attacks after weight loss surgery are not common, but they can occur.

Arrhythmia

Arrhythmias are abnormal heart rates. In an arrhythmia, your heart may beat too fast or too slow, or different parts of your heart may beat independently.

Different medications are available to treat the different kinds of arrhythmias, but sometimes electric-shock therapy is used to convert the rhythm back to normal.

Arrhythmias can be life threatening and require further evaluation. Among severely obese people, arrhythmias can cause sudden death.

Although this may sound frightening, remember that the incidence of sudden death in patients who are severely obese and do *not* undergo surgery is 20 times higher than that of the general population.

Congestive heart failure

Congestive heart failure means that your heart is not pumping as well as it should and there is a backup of fluid. Usually, this means you have difficulty breathing, and you may have swelling of the extremities. Your doctor will give you a medication to make you urinate the extra fluid, and you may get a medication to make your heart beat better.

Respiratory Issues

Respiratory failure means that, for some reason, you aren't breathing well enough on your own. The function of breathing is to get oxygen into your body and carbon dioxide out of your body. Sometimes either you can't get the oxygen in or you can't get rid of the carbon dioxide without the assistance of a *ventilator,* a machine that breathes for you.

During your surgery, you'll be on a ventilator. After you're completely awake from the anesthesia, you'll be taken off the ventilator. If you're having a complication, you may not breathe as well and may need the help of the ventilator until the complication is resolved. If you need to be on the ventilator for more than two weeks, your doctor may perform a *tracheostomy,* which means that the breathing tube will be put through a hole in your trachea in your neck. This is usually temporary, and after the breathing tube is removed, the hole in your trachea and skin closes with a small scar. Some people have such severe sleep apnea that they may require a tracheostomy before their weight loss surgery.

Another possible complication of weight loss surgery is *pneumonia,* which is an infection in your lungs. Pneumonia can occur after any major surgery, and it can show up as fever, cough, and chest pain. Your doctor will order a chest X-ray and/or a chest CAT scan to diagnose this; he'll also take a sample of your phlegm and test it. Antibiotics usually cure pneumonia. You may or may not have to stay in the hospital to start your treatment. In some severe cases, you'll also require a *bronchoscopy,* where a doctor puts a lighted camera down your throat into your trachea and its branches to remove or culture the phlegm.

Infection

Infections can occur with any surgery. In the following sections, we cover two types of infections that occur with weight loss surgery.

Wound infection

Wound infections can occur with open and laparoscopic weight loss surgery (though they're more common with open surgeries). They're more common with gastric bypass, sleeve gastrectomy, and duodenal switch procedures than with gastric banding. This is because the stomach and/or intestines are cut in gastric bypass, sleeve, and duodenal switch, but not in gastric banding.

When an infection occurs, part of the incision usually is opened, and the infection is allowed to drain. You're also started on an antibiotic. Sometimes with an open incision, you have to pack the incision and change the dressings a couple times a day. Depending on the size of the wound and the amount it's opened, a wound infection can take two to four weeks to heal.

Intrabdominal abscess

An *abscess* is basically a collection of pus. Pus is what remains when the cells in your blood that fight infection (the white blood cells) take care of business. An intrabdominal abscess occurs much more commonly with gastric bypass, sleeve gastrectomy, and duodenal switch than it does with gastric banding — and still it occurs in only about 0.5 percent to 1 percent of patients who undergo stapling procedures.

If you have an abscess, you'll be put on antibiotics, and your doctor may need to reoperate to drain the abscess. Or she may have the radiologist drain it with a small catheter that is placed with X-ray guidance. The drains stay in until the abscess cavity gets smaller and the drainage is minimal, which usually also means that the infection is gone. In some cases, you may be treated with antibiotics alone.

Stricture

Stricture is a narrowing caused by scar tissue. Stricture usually occurs at the hookup of the intestine to the new stomach in a gastric bypass, in the hookup of the *duodenum* (the first portion of the small intestine) to the intestine in a duodenal switch, or in the new stomach of a sleeve gastrectomy. Part of healing is scar formation and, basically, when a stricture occurs, your body has healed that hookup or new stomach too much. A stricture usually occurs three weeks to three months after gastric bypass and duodenal switch surgery, but it can occur earlier in a sleeve gastrectomy.

As the hookup or new stomach narrows, you become unable to tolerate solid food and may not be able to tolerate liquids as well. If you're unable to tolerate the same food from one day to the next, this isn't a cause for alarm. However, if you're not able to tolerate *any* food (meaning, you throw up every time you eat), you should call your surgeon.

If you have a stricture, you'll need to have an upper endoscopy done with a dilation. In an upper endoscopy, a lighted camera is put down your throat into your stomach (don't worry — you're usually sedated during this procedure). As the gastroenterologist or surgeon is looking at the narrowed hookup or new stomach, a small balloon is passed across the narrowed area and blown up to gently stretch it open; this is known as *dilation.* This procedure does bring with it some risks, like rupture of the hookup or new stomach, which is why the dilations are done gently. More than one dilation usually is required to get the size of the hookup or new stomach back up to what it was immediately after surgery.

Some gastroenterologists or surgeons may take a look first to see what needs to be done and then schedule the dilation. Most patients need at least two to three dilations to tolerate solid food again.

If you have been vomiting a great deal you may become acutely deficient of vitamin B1 (thiamine). Be sure to let your treating team know so that they can supplement you with an injection.

A stricture also can occur at the hookup of the intestine to the intestine in both duodenal switch and gastric bypass surgery. This stricture usually cannot be dilated because it's much farther downstream and not reachable by endoscopy. If the stricture is at the hookup of the intestine to the intestine, more surgery will be required to fix it.

Dehydration

After you're given the go-ahead to drink following your surgery, be sure to follow your doctor's instructions concerning the amount of fluid you should drink. Your body needs fluid to flush out the waste products and to maintain the body systems.

Initially, you'll struggle to take in all the liquid required, because your pouch has just been formed and it's swollen, leaving very little room for anything. The trick is to sip and sip until you drink your required amount; if you don't drink enough, you could become dehydrated.

Here are some of the signs of dehydration:

✔ Dry mouth

✔ Dark urine

✔ Infrequent urination

✔ Constipation

✔ Lightheadedness

✔ Fainting

Dehydration can worsen your kidney function. It's also a big risk for blood-clot formation. So, you can walk all you want after the surgery, but if you aren't hydrated, you could still form a clot anyway.

 If your surgeon wants you to get in eight 8-ounce glasses (64 ounces) of water or noncaffeinated, noncaloric liquids per day, it's not impossible. Pace yourself by drinking 4 ounces every hour when you're awake. That's only ½ cup per hour, and it's very manageable.

Gastric Prolapse or Band Slippage

With gastric-banding surgery, part of the stomach from below the band can slip through above the band, which results in obstruction and causes you to throw up. Gastric prolapse also can decrease the blood flow to the part of the stomach above the band. You may experience pain or discomfort. Call your surgeon if you're unable to keep even liquids down.

Gastric prolapse occurs in up to 10 percent of patients. It's corrected by another surgery, generally done laparoscopically. During the second surgery, the part of your stomach that slipped above the band is pulled down. Your surgeon may have to remove the band, depending on the condition of your stomach.

Port and Tubing Problems

With the gastric-banding procedure, the port and the tubing can disconnect, break, or leak. If this happens, you lose your restriction and are able to eat a lot more — which isn't a good thing. If the port and tubing disconnect, it's easy to fix but it does mean an outpatient surgery.

Another possible complication is the port flipping on its side. If this happens, filling the band is difficult, or you may experience pain where the port is anchored. The port will need to be repositioned, which also requires an outpatient surgery.

Ulcers

An *ulcer* is a breakdown in tissue. Ulcers usually are related to inflammation. With gastric bypass, ulcers can occur either in the stomach lining of your new pouch or in the intestinal lining, and they're usually located right near the new hookup of your intestine to the stomach. You also may have ulcers in the bypassed stomach and intestine, although that isn't common. With duodenal switch, the ulcers can occur in the stomach, in the duodenum, or in the bypassed duodenum. You can still get ulcers if you have gastric banding; they can be in the stomach above or below the band or in the duodenum. If you have a sleeve gastrectomy, you can get ulcers in the new stomach or in the duodenum.

Ulcers usually cause either pain or nausea and most ulcers can be diagnosed by upper endoscopy. All ulcers are treated with medication to decrease acid production by the stomach, and sometimes with a medication that coats the ulcer as well. If you're experiencing upper-abdominal pain anytime after your surgery, let your surgeon know. An untreated ulcer can lead to more problems, such as bleeding or perforation of the stomach or intestine. Smoking has been strongly linked to ulcers in weight loss surgery patients. Just another reason to quit!

Bowel Obstruction

Any time you have abdominal surgery, you're at risk for bowel obstruction. This is because, when the belly is entered either with an open or laparoscopic approach, your body heals with scar tissue. Scar tissue can form on the inside, and the intestines or bowels can twist around the scar tissue. If this happens, the bowels are blocked, and they back up.

If you have a bowel obstruction, you'll throw up and/or your belly will be bloated. Sometimes, depending on the level of the blockage in your intestine, you may not throw up but you may just have severe abdominal pain. If you experience any of these symptoms, call your surgeon.

You'll have abdominal X-rays performed, including a CAT scan of the abdomen. Depending on your physical exam, you may or may not require surgery. Sometimes by sucking out the fluid that's backing up, the bowel gets a chance to untwist. (The fluid is sucked out by placing a tube up your nose into your stomach pouch and then attaching the tube to suction.) If you require surgery, the procedure may be done laparoscopically or via an open incision. If the bowel has been obstructed for a long time, or if the blood flow to the bowel has been compromised, your doctor may have to take out a piece of your bowel. In some cases, a part of the bowel may have to be brought out on the belly wall with an *ileostomy* (an opening in which part of your intestine is brought up through your belly wall to empty into a bag) or *colostomy* (an opening in which part of your colon is brought up through your belly wall to empty into a bag).

Hernias

There are two types of hernias to watch out for — internal hernias and incisional hernias:

✔ **Internal hernias:** Internal hernias occur when bowel passes under bowel. With gastric bypass and duodenal switch, the rearrangement of the intestines creates a potential trap. Sometimes these traps are closed, but as you lose weight, the traps open again. Signs of an internal hernia are crampy, intermittent abdominal pain and sometimes nausea and vomiting.

If you have an internal hernia, you'll definitely need more surgery to fix it and to pull the intestines out of the trap. Sometimes the blood supply to the bowel can be interrupted as the bowel passes into the trap. If this occurs, some of your bowel may have to be removed.

When your procedure is done laparoscopically, you tend to form less scar tissue, which may result in more internal hernias. The good news is that, if caught early, the surgery to fix the internal hernia also can be done laparoscopically. If the bowel that is trapped has to be removed, the operation may have to be done with a big incision.

✔ **Incisional hernias:** An incisional hernia is a hole in your muscle where the surgeon cut the muscle to perform your surgery. It can occur at any time after your surgery (from hours to years). Some signs of incisional hernias are pain and/or bulging in the area, nausea, and vomiting. Even though your surgeon may have closed the muscle layer at the time of surgery, a weakness or hole can occur. An incisional hernia also requires surgery to be fixed. Sometimes, you'll need a placement of mesh to bolster your muscle, depending on the size of the hernia and the condition of your muscle. The mesh is a synthetic sterile material that is incorporated by your body tissues and lends strength to the closure of your muscle. Incisional hernia repairs can be done with an open or laparoscopic approach.

You may have had surgery prior to your weight loss surgery and have an existing hernia. Your surgeon may or may not close it at the time of the weight loss surgery. Obesity makes you prone to hernias and fixing the hernia before you've lost a significant amount of weight can result in the hernia coming back. In some cases, your surgeon will go ahead and fix an existing hernia at the time of weight loss surgery to prevent the bowel from getting stuck in the hernia.

Esophageal Dilation

Your esophagus is a muscular tube. Sometimes with gastric banding, the esophagus can *dilate,* or lose its shape. This occurs because the muscle of the esophagus is not working properly. When you swallow, a muscular wave propels food into the stomach. When the band is in place, the muscular wave meets a lot of resistance and, in some cases, the esophageal muscle loses some of its tone.

Esophageal dilation is diagnosed by an upper GI series. If you have esophageal dilation, it's usually fixed by pulling some of the fluid out of the band. After anywhere from two to six weeks, your esophagus should regain its muscle tone and contour. With close supervision, the band can be slowly adjusted again.

Pancreatitis

Pancreatitis can occur after duodenal switch surgery. The pancreas lies directly behind the first portion of the small intestine, called the *duodenum.* In the duodenal switch, the duodenum is divided to perform the bypass. The pancreas can become inflamed after the surgery, and this condition is known as *pancreatitis.* Pancreatitis is treated with intravenous nutrition, and you can't eat or drink anything until the inflammation subsides substantially. In some cases, the inflammation is so severe that multiple organs in the body may be affected.

Liver Failure

Liver failure can occur with biliopancreatic diversion with or without duodenal switch. Close follow-up with your surgeon is necessary, and your blood work should be checked every six months after the surgery for the rest of your life. Liver failure can be related to malnutrition; sometimes it can be caught early with close follow-up. Reversal of the intestinal bypass may be necessary if you have liver failure.

Nausea

Nausea right after surgery can be caused by something mechanical (like an obstruction), or it can be related to medications you're getting (for example, many of the pain medications you take after surgery can cause nausea). Sleeve gastrectomy patients can experience more nausea than other weight loss surgery patients. Bear that in mind, and when you leave the hospital ask your surgeon if you should be given anti-nausea medication to take home with you.

In some cases, cessation of antidepressant medications can be associated with nausea. Be sure to restart this medication after you've confirmed with your surgeon that it's safe to do so.

If you have nausea right after the surgery, tell your surgeon. He may change your pain medication to help ease the nausea or add anti-nausea medication.

Comparing risks with other surgeries

Yes, weight loss surgery involves risk, but other surgeries can be just as risky, if not more so. The death rates from heart surgery and colon surgery are approximately 2 percent to 3 percent. And leak rates can be as high as 7 percent following non-bypass gastric surgery. This is significantly higher than with gastric banding, gastric bypass, sleeve gastrectomy, and duodenal switch surgery. So, why all the fuss?

Well, the general public has a different perception about weight loss surgery than heart bypass or colon cancer surgery. They don't think of obesity as a disease — just like heart disease and cancer — but it actually is.

Remember: As with any surgery, risks are involved. You and your doctor have to be sure that the benefits of weight loss surgery outweigh the risks of the surgery *and* the risks of not doing any surgery at all.

Can I take it back?

If you find yourself asking whether the surgery is reversible, you may be overlooking the fact that you have a disease that is genetic, environmental, and social. Weight loss surgery helps, but it only addresses part of the problem. Reversing the weight loss surgery is akin to going off the diet. You'll regain all the weight and then some. Having said that, both the gastric banding and the bypass have been reversed (although not often) because of complications caused by the procedure or because the patient just couldn't tolerate the results of the procedure psychologically. The gastric band can be removed, and the anatomy of the stomach is essentially unchanged. The gastric bypass also can be reversed, but it involves a great deal more surgery than to do it in the first place. The sleeve gastrectomy or biliopancreatic diversion (with or without duodenal switch) cannot be reversed completely, because part of the stomach is removed and will not grow back.

As you get further out from surgery, nausea can be a symptom of many other problems, ranging from minor to major. Here are some of the things that can cause nausea:

- **Certain foods:** Certain foods you eat may cause your nausea — even if you were able to eat the foods and even enjoy them before your surgery. Keep track of what you're eating to get a sense of what may be causing your nausea.

- **Dumping syndrome:** Nausea is a sign of *dumping syndrome* (which happens when you eat foods that are too sweet or too high in fat). See Chapter 18 for more on dumping syndrome.

- **Low blood sugar:** Try eating a cracker. If it helps with your nausea or headache, you need to space your meals better.

- **Ulcers:** Nausea can be a symptom of an ulcer. See "Ulcers," earlier in this chapter.

- **Obstructions:** Nausea can be a sign of a bowel obstruction. See "Bowel Obstruction," earlier in this chapter.

Make sure you let your surgeon know if nausea occurs regularly.

In some cases, nausea can occur for a prolonged time without an apparent cause. If your surgeon is able to rule out more serious problems, she'll prescribe anti-nausea medication to help with your nausea.

Chapter 5

Drafting Your Dream Team: It's More Than a Surgeon

In This Chapter

▶ Selecting a surgeon

▶ Knowing what questions to ask

▶ Taking a look at the rest of the surgical team

*A*fter you decide to have weight loss surgery, one of the more important decisions you'll make will be which surgeon you'll go to for the procedure. You want your surgical experience to be a safe one, and your surgeon is the one person who has more effect on your safety than anyone. In this chapter, we walk you through the process of choosing a surgeon.

As important as surgeons are, they aren't the only ones who affect the success of your surgery. In this chapter, we fill you in on the other important players on your dream team.

Choosing the Right Surgeon for You

Think of your surgeon as the team captain. The surgeon is the team's most important member. Weight loss surgery is only a tool that can help you achieve your weight loss goals, and the surgeon is the one who crafts that tool for you.

As the head of the surgical team, the surgeon holds your life in his hands. The surgeon's skill can literally mean the difference between life and death. Therefore, the selection of a surgeon is a serious one.

In the following sections, we help you come up with a list of surgeons who may be right for you, interview the surgeons to see which one is the best fit, and decide whether issues like geographical distance and a waiting period should be factors in your decision.

Coming up with a list of candidates

Weight loss surgery is also known as *bariatric surgery,* and bariatric surgery is a subspecialty of general surgery. Most bariatric surgeons do other surgeries besides weight loss surgery (for example, they may remove gall bladders or operate on those who have colon cancer). Bariatric surgeons perform an array of surgeries, but you want your surgeon to be experienced with weight loss surgeries — it just makes sense that the more often your surgeon does surgeries like the one you'll be having, the more practice she has, and the better she'll be.

Here are some ways of locating the names of surgeons in your area who perform weight loss surgery:

✔ **Ask your primary-care physician and any of your specialists.** Your doctors have probably had other patients ask the same question. You can collect names from your doctors, but doing your own research and taking everything in this chapter into consideration are critical to your journey. A surgeon's standing in the medical community is important. However, these recommendations from your physicians are only one element in determining who should do your surgery.

✔ **Visit the website of the American Society for Metabolic & Bariatric Surgery (ASMBS;** www.asmbs.org**).** The site lists members by geographic region. It also makes it clear which surgeries each physician performs, whether he sees other surgeons' patients, and so on. (If your surgery is performed elsewhere, you'll need a local surgeon who will do your follow-up.)

✔ **Go to ObesityHelp (**www.obesityhelp.com**), click "Find a Bariatric Surgeon," and search for surgeons in your area.** You can view patient comments here as well. *Remember:* Although these comments can be very helpful, they're just opinions. Bear in mind that this is a commercial site, and if a surgeon pays a high enough fee, negative patient comments can be edited out.

After you have a list of surgeons who may be right for you, you can start evaluating each surgeon and his practice to find the very best fit for your needs.

Asking the right questions

After you have a list of surgeons in your area who perform weight loss surgery, call each office and ask if the surgeon's practice holds free informational or support-group meetings. These meetings are an excellent way to get an introduction to the surgeon, because the surgeon generally will attend.

Check with your state's medical board to find out if the surgeon has been involved in any lawsuits. A lawsuit isn't necessarily a reason to rule out a particular surgeon, but it's something you'll want to ask the surgeon about so you can hear his perspective. Not all licensing boards give out this information, but at the very least they can tell you if there is disciplinary action, which is even more valuable.

You may be put off by a surgeon who has had patients die, but look a little deeper. Some excellent surgeons take on the challenge of operating on very high-risk patients (those who have a very high body mass index and severe health complications going into surgery). These surgeons may be more skilled than those who operate on the more routine cases and have had no deaths.

If you're satisfied with what you've heard at an informational or support-group meeting for a particular surgeon's practice, you're ready to schedule an appointment.

Some surgeons don't hold informational meetings, so just book an appointment for a consultation and take it from there. You may book appointments with several surgeons, but try to attend an informational session if it's offered.

All surgeons should have a support group; this is a good way to see how patients are doing and how they feel about the practice.

The first time you meet individually with the surgeon can be an intimidating experience. You may be frightened by the idea of having surgery, but at the same time, you want the surgeon to be willing to work with you. So questioning a surgeon may be the *last* thing you want to do, for fear of offending her.

Your safety is at stake, so gather your courage and ask away. Be sure to have your questions written down ahead of time, and take a pad of paper with you to write down the surgeon's answers. You also may want to take a family member or friend with you to the appointment; having another set of eyes and ears to catch the things you don't notice or forget is always a bonus.

Here's a list of questions you may want to ask the surgeons you're considering:

✔ **How long have you been doing bariatric surgery?** Find out how much experience the surgeon has with the procedure you want to have.

✔ **How many surgeries have you done?** Studies have shown that the more weight loss procedures a surgeon has performed, the safer his patients are. There is a very definite learning curve in doing bariatric surgery. Surgeons need to start by assisting experienced bariatric surgeons before performing the surgeries on their own. (This experience also can be gained with special training in bariatric surgery known as a *fellowship.*) After a certain number of these assists, the surgeon can then take the lead in surgery with the experienced surgeon assisting.

✔ **Have any of your patients died within 30 days of surgery? If so, what were the circumstances? Were the patients high risk or were the complications just unexplained?** Some very experienced surgeons take on high-risk patients, which sometimes accounts for deaths. The mortality rate for weight loss surgery is ¼ percent to ½ percent.

✔ **Are you board certified?** When a surgeon is board certified, that represents a higher level of proficiency.

✔ **What percentage of your practice is bariatric surgery?** A surgeon should have at least 50 percent of her practice devoted to bariatric surgery. How much of the surgeon's practice is devoted to weight loss surgery is a reflection of how involved the surgeon is with bariatrics.

✔ **What led you to start doing bariatric surgery?** The surgeon's answer will give you an idea of the surgeon's level of commitment to his patients. Was the initial interest because of a technical curiosity in laparoscopy or a sensitivity toward the obese and a desire to help with this disease?

✔ **Are you a member of the American Society for Metabolic & Bariatric Surgery?** The ASMBS is the professional organization for those involved in bariatrics. The surgeon should definitely be a member, as should many of the other members of her practice. The ASMBS is involved in setting standards for bariatric surgery and for hosting educational annual meetings, workshops, and courses for ongoing training.

✔ **How were you trained to do bariatric surgery? Was it a weekend course, special training during a residency, or the completion of a bariatric fellowship?** The more education the better. A weekend course is not enough. A bariatric fellowship is the ideal.

✔ **Do you do surgery laparoscopically?** Surgery done laparoscopically is less invasive and normally involves fewer wound complications, is less painful, and has a quicker recovery time.

✔ **What different types of weight loss surgery do you do and what are your opinions of them?** Most surgeons do more than one kind of surgery, usually the Roux-en-Y gastric bypass, gastric banding, and increasingly the sleeve gastrectomy as well. This will give you options to consider.

✓ **Do you have a surgical team that you always use? If so, how long have you been working together?** A surgical team that has been working together for a year or two can perform surgery faster and more efficiently.

✓ **Will your office help me with insurance approval?** Trying to get your own insurance approval can be a nightmare. If there is someone in the office who specializes in getting insurance approval, your chances of being covered are enhanced.

✓ **Will I have to lose weight prior to surgery?** Some surgeons want patients to lose weight so they'll be healthier going into surgery. Others want a weight loss to show a level of commitment. This is not a negative — but it is something you should know upfront so you're prepared.

✓ **What pain medication will you prescribe while in the hospital and after?** Some patients experience nausea from some pain medication. Other patients require more medication because pain tolerances vary. If you're familiar with how you respond, you can discuss that at the consultation.

✓ **What pretesting will I go through?** Tests allow your surgeon to have a clear picture of your health. For a discussion of pretesting, see Chapter 7.

✓ **How much can my family members be involved during and immediately following my surgery?** Your family members will be your eventual support system. The sooner they're involved, the more support they'll be able to give. If you'd like your family to stay with you while you're in the hospital, find out if accommodations can be made.

✓ **Will you speak to my family following surgery?** Your family will be anxious and concerned. They'll want to hear directly from the surgeon how everything went and be reassured that you're okay or hear what complications you may be experiencing.

✓ **How long a waiting list do you have?** When you decide to have weight loss surgery, you'll probably want to have it right away. But if your ideal surgeon has a waiting list, you may have to wait an additional six months or more for surgery. Sometimes this can be a blessing in disguise. Some insurance plans require documentation of attempts at weight loss. This is the perfect time to do this. Remember also that the reason your doctor's wait time is so long is that he's very competent and in demand. But you'll have to decide if the wait is worth it.

Here are some questions to consider when deciding whether to wait or to go to your runner-up choice:

- **Have you been told by a doctor that you must have the surgery as soon as possible?** If you're in such poor health that waiting is unwise, consider another surgeon. But before you do, make it clear to the surgeon who is your first choice that you've been advised not to wait. Your first-choice surgeon may be able to do something to move you up on the waiting list.

- **How does your first-choice surgeon compare to the other surgeons on your list?** If your first choice is a superior surgeon, and you can safely postpone the surgery, consider waiting. On the other hand, if you feel comfortable that another surgeon is as good as your first choice, select the one with the shorter waiting time — but take into consideration everything in this chapter when coming to that conclusion.

✔ **How often will I have appointments with you after surgery?** Follow-up after surgery is very important. You should expect to see your surgeon after 10 days, 3 weeks, 3 months, 6 months, 9 months, 12 months, 18 months, and then annually if you had gastric bypass or sleeve gastrectomy. If you're having gastric banding surgery, your visits will be at two weeks, and then every month for the first year, every two to three months for the second year, and then every six months. With a duodenal switch, it will be at 2 weeks, 6 weeks, 3 months, 6 months, 9 months, 12 months, and then every 6 months.

✔ **Will you work with my primary-care physician or specialist concerning my care after my surgery?** Make sure the lines of communication are open.

✔ **Is the practice accredited by a national certifying body? If not, why not?** The joint accreditation is a designation given to those practices that meet the highest standards set by the ASMBS and the American College of Surgeons (ACS). If the practice is accredited, it means they've been evaluated and found to provide the equipment and processes that help you have a safe surgical outcome. It also means that the center reports all its data to a registry to keep track of its cases and continuously work to improve its care. It's like having the Good Housekeeping Seal of Approval. You'll have the most comprehensive and best care at these facilities. You may even have the best chance of getting insurance approval. Some insurance companies may require that your surgery be performed at one of these accredited centers. (See the nearby sidebar for more on this important designation.)

✔ **Do you have a support group? If so, do you attend?** Attending a support group is another step toward success. Here you'll meet others who are going through the same things that you'll be going through. Plus, if the surgeon attends, you'll have ready access on a monthly basis to pose to either the surgeon or to someone on the staff any smaller concerns you may have.

ACS/ASMBS accreditation in metabolic and bariatric surgery

If a weight loss surgery program is accredited, you know that the hospital and surgeons are committed to the best patient care and to using their data to continuously strive to improve bariatric surgery. Here are some of the criteria a hospital must meet in order to be awarded this designation:

✔ The hospital must be committed to the medical care of bariatric patients by requiring regular staff training.

✔ The hospital must track its outcomes or do a minimum number of procedures for competency.

✔ There must be a medical director of bariatric surgery.

✔ A full team of specialists must be available for the care of the patient.

✔ The hospital must have appropriately sized equipment and furniture.

✔ The bariatric surgeon must be board certified.

✔ Bariatric surgery must be done following standard procedures.

✔ There must be a designated team involved in the continuing care of patients.

✔ There should be an available support group.

✔ The practice must demonstrate a commitment to patient follow-up.

For more information on the accreditation program go to the website of the ASMBS (www.asmbs.org) or the ACS (www.facs.org).

There is another element to finding the best practice: how the members of the practice make you feel about yourself and about the surgery. The more comfortable you feel, the more inclined you'll be to participate in the all-important after-care program. If you don't like those in the practice, you'll be less likely to go to monthly support-group meetings and keep your appointments, and you'll be less likely to call upon members of the practice for help — all of which will impact your success.

Ask yourself the following questions to get a sense of how comfortable you are with the surgeon and her practice:

✔ **Are the waiting room chairs large enough? Do the chairs have arms?** You've probably sat in chairs much too small for you, but you shouldn't have to endure that in your surgeon's office. The size of the chairs is an indication of the sensitivity toward people of size, and you deserve that in your surgeon's office.

✔ **Does the practice have scales that will weigh in excess of 500 pounds?** Be sure that your weight doesn't exceed the capacity of the scales in your surgeon's office. Your weight will need to be accurately tracked.

✔ **Are your phone calls returned?** You may not have an immediate response, but you should receive a return call within 24 hours.

✔ **Are you generally treated with respect?** Your questions and concerns should be taken seriously, and you should be spoken to with a level of respect. If you're made to feel that your concerns are silly and you're a bother, find another practice.

✔ **Does the surgeon take the time to answer your questions?** Your surgeon will no doubt be busy, but does he have time to answer your questions fully and make you feel like your questions matter? Or is he doing a quick exam and running out the door? You obviously want the former, not the latter.

✔ **Do you feel that the surgeon has a true concern about her patients and about you?** Go with your instincts on this one. Does your surgeon exhibit care? What do the other patients have to say? Strike up conversations in the waiting room and at support-group meetings. Other patients will give you a good idea of what you can expect.

✔ **Is your spouse, partner, or close friend welcome to ask questions and attend group meetings and appointments?** You want a surgeon who is receptive to questions from your family members and friends. They're the people who will be your support system, and they need a lot of information to help you.

All these questions count and will have an impact upon your choice and upon your success. *Remember:* You and your surgeon should feel like a good fit.

The way to find your perfect fit is to shop around. You can get a good feel for a practice by visiting and asking questions. You'll get a sense for how you're treated and have your specific questions answered. You can attend not only the informational meetings but support-group meetings as well. Visit as many practices as you feel necessary.

The Supporting Players

Your choice of surgeon is important for your safety, but of equal or even greater importance in your long-term success are those members of the team who will provide you with support prior to your surgery, be involved with your actual surgery, and guide you during your after-care. These members are part of the practice team that the surgeon has to offer. This section introduces you to the people who may be on your team.

Psychologist

You'll first meet the psychologist during your pre-op testing. The psychologist will administer a psychological evaluation prior to surgery. Often the psychologist will attend support-group meetings. She should have extensive experience working with those who have weight problems, as well as with weight loss surgery patients.

In the period following surgery, the psychologist can be especially helpful. Following surgery, you may go through a period of depression as you realize what you've done. Then your body realizes that you aren't going to be eating as you ate before. This often triggers another round of depression. You'll also have body-image issues to deal with. Problems with family members and friends may crop up as you're changing so rapidly. And eating issues are often still there even after weight loss surgery. A psychologist can help with all these issues.

Dietitian

A dietitian can be an invaluable asset following your surgery. You'll be learning a new way of eating — not just for the first year, but for a lifetime — and your dietitian should be there to guide you along the way. Find out from the dietitian what his level of experience is with weight loss surgery patients. The more experience, the better.

You should be given a series of menus for the first several weeks. Review them with the dietitian and ask any questions you may have. You also should discuss a vitamin regimen, which is vital to your health. You want to make sure you understand everything the dietitian tells you, because this information will form the basis of a new healthy lifestyle.

Bariatric coordinator

A bariatric coordinator is the person you'll consult with for general questions before and after surgery. Often, she's the person who runs the support group. This is the person on the other end of the phone when you're in a panic over your insurance coverage or over a detail following your surgery.

The bariatric coordinator needs general knowledge about surgery and its aftermath. She needs to be a good communicator, organized, patient, and compassionate. Often, you just need reassurance that everything is all right — in these situations, the bariatric coordinator is the one who will hold your hand.

Traveling for surgery

You may consider traveling outside your area for weight loss surgery, but think very carefully before you take this step.

Here are some valid reasons to travel for surgery:

✔ **You don't have a good bariatric surgeon in your area.** If your only option is to have surgery done by a surgeon who does very few weight loss surgeries per year, or if your community has no bariatric surgeon, you'll have to travel outside your area.

✔ **You have severe health problems and have no family or friends in your area.** If you know of a good practice in another area where you have family and friends you can move in with, consider traveling for surgery. Only do this if you'll be staying with your family or friends for an extended period of time; otherwise, investigate rehabilitation facilities that are available in your own area. The facility will help to fill in the support you're lacking at home.

Here are some situations in which you *wouldn't* want to travel to have your surgery done:

✔ **You have a very good bariatric surgeon in your area.** If that's the case, don't consider going to another surgeon far away because you think she may be better. The after-care services you'll miss out on locally aren't worth the trip.

✔ **You aren't covered by insurance and you've exhausted all appeals, so you're considering having the surgery performed outside the United States where it's less expensive.** Research these centers very carefully and tour them beforehand. Make sure the center is well equipped to take care of all potential problems. *Note:* If you travel out of the country for surgery, you may have difficulty finding a surgeon in the United States who will treat you if you encounter complications after you've returned home.

Bariatrician

Also on staff at your surgeon's office may be a bariatrician. This is a physician who has received special ongoing and extensive training in issues of obesity and related conditions. Bariatricians are members of the American Society of Bariatric Physicians (ASBP; www.asbp.org).

Bariatricians play different roles from one practice to the next. The bariatrician may be the person who initially determines that you've really worked at dieting. He may work with you for a few months prior to surgery to assure your insurance company you're unable to effectively lose weight by dieting. A bariatrician can be a focal point for your weight loss journey after your surgery, by monitoring your weight loss, helping to direct you regarding exercise, and assisting you in maintaining your weight loss for years down the road.

Part II
Preparing for Surgery

The 5th Wave   By Rich Tennant

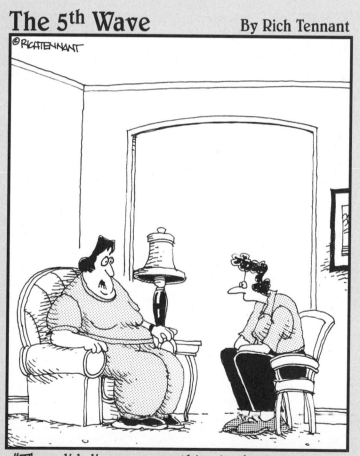

"They did discover something in the pre-surgery physical that I'm afraid came as a surprise to me. Apparently, I have a tattoo of a bumblebee over my right butt cheek with the nickname 'Honey Buns' written underneath."

In this part . . .

Most often, weight loss surgery is paid for by insurance, but you must meet certain qualifications in order to be covered. In this part, we tell you when a "no" from your insurance company doesn't really mean "no" and show you how to handle an appeal if it becomes necessary.

Your first goal with weight loss surgery will be to get through the operation as safely as possible. You'll be required to undergo numerous tests so your surgeon has an accurate picture of the state of your health going into surgery; in this part, we tell you what to expect. We also fill you in on the importance of physical exercises and breathing exercises that will make your recovery easier. Finally, we tell you what you should take care of at home before your trip to the operating room, so you can focus on your recovery instead of on household chores.

Chapter 6

Paying for Surgery: No Assurance of Insurance

• •

In This Chapter

▶ Understanding the requirements

▶ Appealing if you're denied insurance coverage

▶ Paying for surgery yourself

• •

*O*ne of the first considerations that may have come to mind when you started thinking about weight loss surgery is, "How am I going to pay for it?" If you have health insurance, that's not necessarily a guarantee that weight loss surgery is covered. Even if it is covered, you may have to cross certain hurdles and provide documentation that your insurance company requires for approval.

In this chapter, we let you know how to deal with your insurance company, how to get your physicians' support, and what to do if your insurance company says no. We also give you some options for paying for the surgery out of your pocket, letting you know some of the challenges involved.

Figuring Out What Kind of Coverage You Have

Before you start to worry about how you'll pay for the surgery or how you'll battle with your insurance company, you need to know exactly what your policy covers and what it doesn't.

You're responsible for providing your surgeon with as much information as possible and for having a thorough understanding of your insurance policy. Each company has its own authorization requirements, and each policy is different.

Start by calling your insurance carrier or benefits office. Find out if your policy covers weight loss surgery, and make sure to ask whether there are any exceptions. Also, find out whether the surgeon and hospital you want to use are covered under your policy, or whether you may have to pay at least some of the costs involved if you go with that surgeon or hospital. (See the nearby sidebar, "The major categories of insurance policies," for information on the different kinds of policies and what they typically require.)

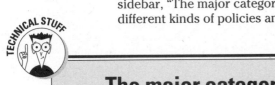

The major categories of insurance policies

Insurance policies known as health maintenance organizations (HMOs) will require you to see a provider who participates in their network. If you're a participant in an HMO plan, you'll need to use your insurance carrier's provider directory to locate a participating provider. You also may want to conduct some online research to help you choose a surgeon who is a member of the plan.

Preferred provider organizations (PPOs) or point of service (POS) plans, allow you to see either an in-network or out-of-network surgeon. If you choose a surgeon in the insurance company's network, you won't have to pay as much money as you will if you choose a surgeon who is out of network. If you choose an out-of-network surgeon, contact your insurance company or benefits office and inquire about any deductible, co-insurance, and out-of pocket maximums that apply to your policy.

Traditional insurance policies have no preferred network of providers. However, you have to pay a larger portion of your healthcare costs. You usually have an annual deductible to meet, after which you have a co-insurance and often an annual out-of-pocket maximum. The benefit of this plan is the flexibility to choose any surgeon and get the same amount of coverage.

The federal government is the largest insurer in the United States, through the Medicare and Medicaid programs. In 2004, Medicare announced that it would remove barriers to covering obesity-related illnesses. With this new policy, Medicare has reviewed scientific evidence in order to determine which interventions improve health outcomes for those Americans who are obese and/or have many of obesity's associated medical conditions. However, Medicare also indicated that there is not enough data to say that weight loss surgery is of proven benefit in the population over 65, which is Medicare's majority coverage. As of this writing, Medicare does not cover sleeve gastrectomy, but that policy is being reviewed in June 2012.

The technicalities of insurance can be difficult — not to mention mind numbing — to navigate. For a great primer on different kinds of medical insurance, and to make sense of the policy you currently have, check out *Insurance For Dummies,* 2nd Edition, by Jack Hungelmann (Wiley).

Nearly all the larger insurance carriers now have written treatment guidelines or policy bulletins for weight loss surgery. Ask where you can find this information on the company's website, or ask the company to send you a copy of these guidelines. Bring a copy of these documents to your appointment with your surgeon; the documents will outline your insurance carrier's requirements for precertification, as well as all the types of surgery that are covered by your policy. Although most companies that cover weight loss surgery approve gastric bypass and gastric banding, not all companies cover sleeve gastrectomy or the biliopancreatic diversion with duodenal switch.

Guidelines for precertification vary from carrier to carrier. Today, most insurance companies require evidence of the *multidisciplinary-team approach* to your surgical treatment. This means that your insurance company wants to see that there is a team of healthcare professionals participating in both your pre- and post-operative care.

If you've changed insurance carriers in the past year, ask whether there is a waiting period on your policy for preexisting conditions. Certain policies will not cover treatment of conditions that are specified as preexisting until a set period of time has passed (for example, six months or a year). This is also referred to as an exclusion for preexisting condition. Your obesity may fall into this category of preexisting conditions; if it does, you can find out exactly what your insurance company will cover and when. Then you can plan your surgery accordingly.

Giving Your Insurance Company the Information It Requires

One of the happiest moments in your weight loss surgery journey is when you get the seal of approval from your insurance company.

Most insurance companies realize the long-term effects and cost savings associated with the weight loss that occurs after patients have weight loss surgery. For example, if you have diabetes, your insurance company will spend thousands of dollars covering your medications and treatment. Paying for one gastric-bypass procedure is likely less expensive for the insurance company than paying for your diabetes medications and treatment for the rest of your life (not to mention paying for any other complications that may arise down the road as a result of your obesity).

Unfortunately, obtaining insurance approval is not always easy. Acquiring insurance coverage for weight loss surgery can be a major obstacle to finally achieving a healthier body and life. Over the past few years, insurance carriers have seen a significant increase in the demand for weight loss surgery procedures. According to the American Society for Metabolic & Bariatric Surgery (ASMBS), 16,200 weight loss procedures were performed in 1994. Fast-forward to today, and approximately 150,000 weight loss surgery procedures are performed annually. The average cost for surgery is now up to approximately $30,000. Due to this increase in procedures and cost, some insurance companies are making it more difficult for patients to obtain approval. These insurance companies don't view their policyholders as long-term responsibilities and figure their customers will switch carriers before they can recoup their investment.

So, what hurdles will you have to cross? Most companies require what's called a *letter of medical necessity* from your bariatric surgeon and your primary-care physician. The following information is generally what's required in this preauthorization letter:

- Your height, weight history, and body mass index (BMI)
- A description of your obesity-related health conditions, including records of treatment
- A detailed description of the limitations your obesity places on your daily activities
- A detailed history of the results of your dieting efforts, including medically and non-medically supervised programs
- A history of exercise programs, including receipts for memberships in health clubs

Ask your doctor to include information from medical journals regarding the effectiveness of weight loss surgery, especially information demonstrating the control or elimination of obesity-related health conditions.

Many carriers also require a nutritional consult and psychological evaluation. Your surgeon will take care of referring you for these consultations.

A number of carriers now require detailed documentation of participation in a physician-supervised diet. Most require the submission of at least six months' worth of office notes from the supervising physician, including proof of dietary supervision and recorded weigh-ins.

Not all primary-care physicians support weight loss surgery. Your physician may not be up to speed on the latest techniques and safety reports; he may be familiar only with older procedures that had higher risks. Don't be discouraged. You can bring information to your doctor to try to change his opinion. If your primary-care physician can't be persuaded, you may have to find another primary-care doctor who understands the necessity for your surgery.

Request letters and documentation from any medical professionals who treated you for health-related conditions caused by or aggravated by obesity. Make sure all the letters are sent directly to you (as opposed to your doctor's office), so you can determine if they're supportive of your case. Be sure to make copies of the letters for your records. In addition, forward to your surgeon anything that documents difficulties related to severe obesity such as:

- High blood pressure
- Diabetes
- Cardiovascular disease
- Sleep apnea
- Gastroesophageal reflux
- Infertility
- Arthritis
- *Dyslipidemia* (a disease characterized by a high concentration of lipids and cholesterol in the blood, a risk factor for heart disease and cardiovascular disease)
- Urinary stress incontinence
- Other obesity-related conditions

Other important information to provide your surgeon includes

- Your weight history, demonstrating a history of severe obesity
- Your current medications
- Your psychiatric history
- Your musculoskeletal history, like joint pain, bone fractures, and osteoarthritis
- Any allergies you have

Each weight loss surgeon's practice has its own way of managing financial and insurance issues. Someone in the office should be able to talk to you about your insurance concerns and questions. Most of these advisors are familiar with the ins and outs of working with specific carriers.

Being familiar with your own policy is still important. Even the most well-informed advisor won't know all the details of your specific policy without some investigation.

Following Up with Your Insurance Company

About a week after your surgeon's office has submitted your forms and letters, contact your insurance company to make sure all the paperwork has been received. Confirm that it has all the necessary information required to render a decision on your surgery.

Before calling, have on hand:

- ✔ Your insurance policy number
- ✔ The exact name of the procedure you're having (for example, Roux-en-Y gastric bypass)
- ✔ Your surgeon's name
- ✔ The name of the hospital where the procedure will be performed

Each time you speak to someone at your insurance company, document the following:

- ✔ The date you called
- ✔ The phone number you dialed
- ✔ The name of the person you spoke with
- ✔ Accurate notes on the conversation you had

Make photocopies of all paperwork you send to your insurance company. Thirty days is the standard time for an insurance provider to respond to your request. If you haven't received a response within that time frame, call and follow up.

A free source of information when dealing with insurance companies can be found at www.obesityaction.org/educational-resources/brochures-and-guides/oac-insurance-guide which walks you through the insurance process and gives you tips if you're denied. The guide includes a sample appeal letter in case you're denied.

Knowing What to Do If You're Denied

Some insurance companies will automatically deny weight loss surgery even if it's medically necessary. Providing additional information is all that's required for approval. Some insurance carriers will continue to say no or insist that you provide them with even more information. They may hope that patients will get frustrated and give up — but not you!

Your health is far too important not to continue to fight for your coverage. If your insurance company continues to request additional information, keep providing it. Also, continue to follow up with the company and make sure you stay on top of the documentation every step of the way.

Some insurance carriers do exclude the treatment of severe obesity from their plans. Many patients see the word *exclusion* and give up. But "no" is not always the final answer. Your employer may be able to purchase a policy for you that covers weight loss surgery. **Remember:** This is your health, and you're paying a lot of money to these companies. You're worth fighting for!

Fighting back

The denial phone call or letter can be devastating, but it's not always the end of the line. Many companies offer the option of an appeal. This can be done within the insurance company or by an outside agency. However, be aware that there are time constraints associated with appeals — you can file an appeal only within a certain time period. In addition, you're allowed only a certain number of appeals — you can't keep appealing forever. Sometimes going to an external appeal is a good idea — your case will be referred to a bariatric surgeon who understands the benefits of weight loss surgery.

If you're denied coverage, your next step is to write an appeal letter. In your letter, make sure you emphasize how weight loss surgery will diminish your obesity-related weight problems. Do *not* say that you're having surgery just to lose weight. You also want to include the following information:

- Your name, height, and weight
- Your BMI along with an explanation of what BMI is (see Chapter 2)
- What you've done to try to lose weight on your own (for example, diets, medications, exercises) and the outcomes (such as weight loss and weight regain)
- All your health problems associated with your obesity
- Any medications you're currently taking
- The length of time you've been overweight
- The social effects of your obesity
- Job-related problems due to your obesity
- Any difficulty you have in doing normal, everyday activities
- Any psychological issues related to your obesity (for example, depression or low self-esteem)

Following the paper trail

Proving that your weight loss surgery is a medical necessity begins with your medical history. One of the top reasons patients get denied by their insurance companies is because they don't have enough documentation demonstrating medical necessity. The more documentation you have to support you, the harder it is for an insurance carrier to deny your claim. So, the minute you begin to contemplate weight loss surgery, have your weight documented by your primary-care physician.

If you've attended a commercial weight-loss program (such as Weight Watchers), try to obtain these records. The records will demonstrate that you *have* made diet attempts. Some insurance companies may allow this as a substitution for a medically monitored diet.

Notes from your visit with the surgeon, your psychological and nutritional evaluations, as well as a letter of support from your primary-care physician, almost always are required. Additional requirements depend on your individual carrier and can include other tests such as a sleep study or thyroid function testing.

After initial receipt of the standard forms and paperwork from your surgeon's office, some insurance companies may request additional proof of dieting. This can include receipts you may have from weight loss medications or diet supplements. Also, providing pictures showing you at various weights, when you've dieted and then regained weight, can be helpful.

Seeking outside help

If you and your surgeon have thoroughly reviewed your denied procedure, you've filed an appeal, and your insurance company remains unmoved, you do have other options.

You can get help from your employer. Contact your benefits coordinator and inform him of the situation. Your employer often can dispute a lack of coverage for something for which the employer is paying to have included in the company's coverage.

If your employer is self-insured and uses third-party administrators to manage its claims, you can appeal directly to your employer. If your employer supports you, it can accept financial responsibility, giving you bariatric surgery benefits.

Other options include switching insurance companies. Employers sometimes offer a choice of insurance companies, or you can purchase your own policy. Just make sure your new company and policy cover weight loss surgery.

If you decide to retain an attorney for your appeal, you may want to contact the Obesity Law and Advocacy Center (www.obesitylaw.com). The firm, which has extensive experience with insurance law, is run by Walter Lindstrom, who is a weight loss surgery patient.

Don't cancel your existing policy until you have proof of insurance in hand from the new company, or you may end up uninsured.

If you do switch insurance companies, be aware that some insurers may consider obesity a preexisting condition and won't cover the surgery in your first six months or year of owning the policy. (Be sure to ask how long you would have to wait.)

You may choose to have your appeal handled by an attorney experienced in insurance law. Such legal tactics have helped numerous patients receive benefits and, ultimately, their surgery, but hiring an attorney is reserved for the appeal.

Paying for Surgery out of Your Own Pocket

If you've exhausted all your insurance options, you may decide to pay for the surgery yourself. You can use a number of financial strategies to pay for weight loss surgery. The first thing you should do is speak with an accountant. Be sure you can afford the surgery and any potential complications that may be associated with it.

Make sure your surgeon will accept you as a patient. Some surgeons will turn away patients who aren't covered under insurance because of the liability involved. If your surgeon accepts self-payment, see if you can negotiate a better rate with the surgeon, the hospital, and the anesthesiologist. Find out if they'll honor the same rate that an insurance company would pay — this rate is usually far less then what you're typically billed. Also, see if the surgeon will be willing to work out a payment schedule with you. Spreading out your payments may make it easier for you than having to pay in one lump sum.

Some surgeons have an arrangement with the insurance company BLIS (www.bliscompany.com), which will provide you with insurance to cover complications following surgery. (It's the complications that can bankrupt you.) Not all surgeons have this arrangement, so check with your surgeon.

Unless you're Donald Trump, you'll probably find paying for your own surgery an expensive undertaking. Possible complications may require additional operations and a longer hospital stay, which can quickly add up to tens of thousands of dollars in hospital bills — and financial ruin. You may want to speak with an accountant before doing this.

Most hospitals and surgeons will accept payment by credit card if you have a high enough credit limit. Keep in mind that putting your surgery on a credit card is not always the best way to finance it, particularly if your card charges high interest rates. You may benefit by checking out these other options:

- **Home equity loan:** If you own a home, a home equity loan may be your best option. The payments may be tax-deductible. The laws in some states dictate that a home equity loan may be used only for home improvements. Make sure you're aware of your mortgage company's policy and your state's laws regarding this option.

- **Bank loan:** If you can get approval, the interest rates on a bank loan are usually lower than they are for credit cards or finance companies.

- **Finance companies:** Finance companies offer loans for your surgery similar to financing a car loan. Make sure you shop around to get the best rates. Ask your surgeon's office if they can recommend a good company.

- **Flexible spending accounts (FSAs):** If your employer offers this benefit, sign up. An FSA allows you to set aside pre-tax dollars to pay for medical expenses not covered by insurance. The amount you can put into this account is set by your employer but usually is several thousand dollars. You must designate the total amount for the year that will be put into this account. The money is then deducted from your pay every pay period. You may then apply to have your medical expenses reimbursed.

  Any money left in your flexible spending account that hasn't been reimbursed is divided among all the participants in your employer's plan. So, don't set aside more money than you're sure you'll need.

- **Financing through your surgeon's office:** A few bariatric programs offer financing for patients who meet the requirements. Check with the financial advisor at your surgeon's office to see if your surgeon offers these services.

You may want to consider a combination of these options.

Regardless of how you pay for your surgery, the expenses may be tax deductible. Consult an accountant before claiming any deduction.

Chapter 7

Making the Grade: Testing Prior to Surgery

· ·

In This Chapter

▶ Identifying which tests you'll need

▶ Understanding why these tests are important

▶ Knowing what your doctor is looking for

· ·

*P*rior to weight loss surgery, you'll undergo major testing. Your medical team needs to make sure you're in the best possible condition before you have major surgery — your surgeon shouldn't be facing any surprises during surgery, so she needs an accurate assessment of your condition.

If you're like many people facing weight loss surgery, you may not have seen a doctor for a while because you were embarrassed about your weight. You may have avoided seeing a doctor because, after all, what would the doctor tell you? Lose weight. As if you didn't know that already.

If you haven't been seen by a doctor in a while, you may find out that you have a few conditions that require some treatment. The most common medical problems in the severely obese are high blood pressure, diabetes, and sleep apnea. It isn't uncommon for patients to discover conditions that they didn't even know they had.

Some of the tests you'll undergo are required by your insurance company, some are required by your surgeon, some are required by your primary-care physician, and some are required by the hospital where your surgery will take place. In this chapter, we give you a rundown of what tests you can expect prior to surgery and why your medical team wants you to have them. Depending on your family or personal health history, you also may have to undergo routine health-screening tests such as a mammogram and pap smear (for women) or a prostate exam (for men).

Psychological Evaluation

Almost everyone who wants to have weight loss surgery has to undergo a psychological evaluation. Some insurance companies and weight loss surgeons require their patients to undergo this evaluation, but check first — some don't require it. The exam includes answering questions and being evaluated by a psychologist.

Sometimes the evaluation includes the Minnesota Multiphasic Personality Inventory (MMPI), which provides an objective personality assessment.

Your surgeon will probably refer you to a mental-health professional — a psychiatrist, psychologist, or social worker — who's familiar with weight loss surgery, the risks involved, and the adjustments you'll need to make after the surgery. *Note:* This evaluation may not be covered by insurance.

Why is a psychological evaluation important, and what is your surgeon looking for? Here are some questions the surgeon will want to be answered in your evaluation:

- ✔ **Are you depressed and, if so, how seriously?** Following surgery, you'll face some difficult times. As the anesthesia and painkillers wear off, you may find yourself depressed. You'll also likely experience depression as your body goes into mourning over the loss of food. And you'll likely experience depression during the long months of adjusting to a new way of eating and when you're having problems with food issues. If your depression is severe going into surgery, your surgeon will want a mental-health professional to diagnose that, so the surgeon can determine whether you'll be able to handle these added issues.

    Most patients who qualify for weight loss surgery show signs of depression. Many are medicated; others are not. If you're depressed, the psych evaluation helps identify the severity of your depression and also identifies the goals and expectations you have for your surgery. Weight loss is not designed to cure depression. It does improve your physical health, which may very well impact your mental health.

- ✔ **Are you suicidal?** If your depression is so severe that you're suicidal, the additional adjustment following surgery will be too difficult for you to endure until you can be successfully treated with mental-health intervention. When you're successfully treated for your mental condition, you'll be reevaluated to determine if you're a good candidate.

- ✔ **How well will you cope after the surgery?** What are the coping mechanisms and potential stress-management techniques you can use after the surgery? Many people who are severely obese have long turned to food as a coping mechanism in time of stress or depression. If you don't have other coping mechanisms in place — including a strong support system of family or friends — you may be inclined to turn immediately to food as your coping mechanism, which will sabotage your surgery or make you very sick.

✔ **Will you be able to comply with post-op restrictions and instructions?** Immediately after surgery, noncompliance with your surgeon's instructions can cause numerous dangerous results, ranging from minor health problems to death. Therefore, your ability to comply with your doctor's orders is extremely important. *Remember:* If you don't take the vitamins your doctor has asked you to take, you may eventually face nutritional deficiencies.

✔ **Do you have a psychiatric disorder or addiction that may impair your judgment?** Are you bulimic or addicted to drugs? Do you have uncontrolled bipolar disorder? Any of these disorders or similar ones can lead to harmful eating behaviors that can jeopardize your health after surgery.

✔ **Are you competent to make the decision to have this surgery?** Weight loss surgery is major surgery, and your surgeon will want to be sure you're able to understand the risks and you've decided, with a sound mind, to have the surgery.

✔ **What kind of support system do you have to help you after the surgery?** If you have a strong support system of family and friends who are aware of what weight loss surgery entails and are prepared to support you every step of the way, you're off to a great start. On the other hand, if you have family and friends who will try to jeopardize your efforts to be healthy through eating and exercise, you need to be aware of it and try to find other avenues of support — *before* your surgery.

The psychological evaluation is valuable for your surgeon *and* for you. Don't try to trick the evaluator. Lying during this evaluation can only hurt you.

Most people could use a little therapy. Food may long have been your best friend, solace, and comfort, and when you can no longer rely on it for support, you need to have another support system in place. A mental-health professional who is familiar with weight loss surgery and with whom you connect is also a possible ally for your short-term and long-term recovery. Don't hesitate to find a therapist *before* your surgery who will be there for you to draw on in the weeks and months *after* your surgery.

Nutritional Evaluation

You've probably dieted for years, and you may even know so much about nutrition that you could write a book. Why do *you* need to see a dietitian?

Well, denial is a part of recovery. A dietitian identifies the type of eating behavior you have. She can instruct you on the major changes you need to make after surgery. As you describe your eating pattern and verbalize your relationship with food, you help to identify potential danger zones after the surgery.

Most people turn to food for support, stress relief, comfort, and many other reasons. Right after the surgery, your emotional or situational triggers can't be relieved with large quantities of food.

Your surgeon will refer you to a dietitian who is familiar with weight loss surgery patients. This person is a valuable source of information for what you can expect and the amount of food you can eat after surgery. She has a wealth of information on what other patients have experienced with their diets. So, be sure to pay attention during this evaluation. The dietitian will give you helpful tips on what types of food to eat throughout the entire course of your recovery. She can help identify good sources of protein for each stage of your recovery. She also can tell you how to eat after the surgery, how much to chew, and what to avoid.

With time, you may be able to eat more and turn to food for all the wrong reasons. A dietitian can help not only with therapy but with good food choices and eating behavior tricks to prevent yourself from regaining weight after your surgery. The bottom line with weight loss surgery is that healthy choices keep your caloric intake to a minimum, and this is an important component of maintaining your weight loss.

When you reach a plateau in your weight loss, the dietitian may have tips on how to kick-start your weight loss again. Keep a food log for several days and be perfectly honest. Include the foods you ate, how much you ate, and the time you took to eat it. Go over this with your dietitian and identify areas that need work. *Remember:* You're a work in progress, and you should call in consultants when you need them.

Blood Work

You didn't think you'd be able to enter the operating room without letting your doctors take some of your blood, did you? Your medical team wants to make sure you're ready for surgery, and your blood tells them a lot about your body and your health.

Which blood tests they'll perform depends on your medical history and sometimes on your family history. Some common tests include the following:

- **Complete blood count (CBC):** The CBC tells your doctors whether you have an infection or are anemic. Anemia is an iron deficiency, and it can be caused by several factors. Newly diagnosed anemia has to be fully evaluated before weight loss surgery, because iron-deficiency anemia is a possibility after weight loss surgery. Your surgery may be postponed until your anemia is fully evaluated by your primary-care doctor and sometimes by a *hematologist* (blood specialist). If you have anemia with a known cause, your surgery may happen as planned. If your anemia responds to iron supplements, your surgeon will want your blood count to be maximized before surgery.

✔ **Metabolic panel:** This test shows how well your body is absorbing nutrients, how well your kidneys are functioning, and how well your liver is working. These are just general indicators that give your doctor an idea of how your body is doing in broad terms — they aren't specific to any particular disease.

✔ **Liver function tests:** As the name implies, these tests measure different aspects of your liver, how the bile is draining, and how healthy your liver tissue is. Some liver abnormalities can be related to cirrhosis or hepatitis. Abnormalities also can be related to fatty liver. Most severely obese patients have *fatty liver,* which means that the liver has excessive fat deposits within the liver tissue. As you lose weight, fatty liver can improve.

Another condition related to fatty liver called nonalcoholic steatohepatitis (NASH) can progress to cirrhosis and end-stage liver disease. Weight loss surgery can reverse some of the changes in the liver associated with NASH.

✔ **Prothrombin time (PT) or partial thromboplastin time (PTT):** These tests measure how well your blood clots. Depending on your medical or family history, these tests and others that check how well your blood clots may or may not be required.

✔ **Hemoglobin A1C:** Along with a fasting blood glucose test, hemoglobin A1C measures how well controlled your diabetes is. Some surgeons may not want to operate if your diabetes is poorly controlled.

✔ **Free T4, thyroid stimulating hormone (TSH):** This test measures your thyroid function. If you have a hypothyroid (low-thyroid) condition, you can gain weight. Obviously, your doctor wants to treat any causes of weight gain that he can.

Your doctor may order other tests. The ones we list here are just some of the most common.

Urinalysis

Yes, your doctor will send you into the bathroom and ask you to pee in a cup. He'll then send your urine for urinalysis, which — you guessed it — is an analysis of your urine. (Aren't doctors a creative group?) Here's what your doctor will be looking for in the urinalysis:

✔ Pregnancy

✔ Infections

✔ Complications of diabetes

✔ Nicotine

Not all doctors test for nicotine in the urine, but some do. If your doctor discovers that you're still smoking, she may refuse to operate. Smoking will adversely affect your respiratory functions (how well you breathe) and your ability to heal by preventing oxygen from getting to all parts of your body. You're at enough risk being severely obese — you don't want to add the risks of smoking to that.

Cardiac Tests

Before you have weight loss surgery, your surgeon will want to be sure that your heart is in tiptop shape. The only way to be sure of your heart's health is to perform some tests, which we cover in the following sections.

Electrocardiogram

Everyone who undergoes weight loss surgery has an electrocardiogram (EKG) beforehand. The EKG lets your doctor know the following:

- **How fast your heart beats:** Your heart can beat at a normal rate or too fast or slow. If it beats too fast or too slow, you'll need more testing to figure out why.

- **Whether the rhythm is normal:** A normal rhythm is called a *sinus rhythm*. If you don't have a sinus rhythm, you'll be evaluated to see if you need further treatment for your heart rhythm before you have any surgery.

- **Whether your heart muscle is working normally:** The EKG allows your doctor to see if the parts of your heart are contracting in the correct sequence. If they aren't, you may need further treatment.

- **Whether your heart muscle has been damaged by a heart attack:** If you've had a heart attack, many times there will be changes on the EKG that alert your doctor to this fact. Having had a heart attack puts you at a higher risk for surgery; you'll definitely undergo more testing.

- **Whether your heart muscle has been working too hard:** The EKG will show if one part of your heart muscle is working harder than the rest of your heart. Usually this indicates that you have high blood pressure. In some cases, this buildup of heart tissue in one part of your heart can lead to other problems that have to be treated before surgery.

- **If there are any changes since the last study:** Your doctor will be able to compare your EKGs and see if you had any silent heart problems. Again, this identifies whether you're at high risk for surgery.

Additional testing

Some people won't need any cardiac testing beyond the EKG. Others — because of their medical history, their family history, or their doctor's preferences — will need one or more additional tests. We cover these in the following sections.

Echocardiogram

An echocardiogram is an ultrasound of your heart. It allows the doctor to determine how well your heart muscle is pumping, how well your heart valves work, and whether your heart muscle is normal or too thick.

If you took the weight loss drug Phen-Fen for more than three months, you may be required to have an echocardiogram if you haven't already had one. Prolonged use of Phen-Fen has been associated with valve problems in some people.

You also may have a heart murmur and, depending on the type of murmur, the echocardiogram can tell your doctor whether the murmur requires treatment. Some heart murmurs are benign; other murmurs require either medication or special management around the time of the surgery by the anesthesiologist and the surgeon.

Stress test

Your doctor may require a stress test to see how well your heart holds up to stress. Why? Because surgery can be stressful on your heart, and your surgeon wants to be sure your heart can tolerate this type of stress.

Not everyone has a stress test prior to surgery — your medical history, family history, and activity level may not necessitate it. However, some doctors require all their weight loss surgery patients to have a stress test, regardless of their history or activity level.

There are two types of stress tests:

- ✔ **Exercise or treadmill stress test:** In this test, you walk on a treadmill, and the doctor looks at what you and your heart do under the stress of exercise.
- ✔ **Medical stress test:** In this test, you're injected with a drug that causes your heart to work harder, inducing a situation similar to what your body would experience if you were on the treadmill.

If you're able to walk on a treadmill, your doctor will probably have you do that. But if you have mobility problems that would prevent you from walking long enough for the test to tell the doctor what he needs to know, he may opt for the medical stress test instead.

Angiogram

You may need an angiogram (sometimes called a *cardiac catheterization*) before your weight loss surgery. An angiogram is the most invasive of all the cardiac tests. A needle and catheter are put into one of your major arteries and the catheter is guided up to your heart so the smaller arteries that bring oxygen to your heart can be outlined on an X-ray.

If you have a significant blockage in one or more of these arteries, you may require new medications, stents to open up the blockage, or heart surgery to bypass the blockage. A stent is placed in the artery to open up the artery and keep it open; placement of the stent is performed by a cardiologist.

Because of the invasiveness of the angiogram, some risks are involved. If you require an angiogram, your cardiologist will outline the risks for you. But remember: The test can provide accurate and lifesaving information.

Pulmonary Tests

A number of lung problems are common in severely obese people. If you're severely obese, you probably find yourself short of breath with activity — this is because your lungs don't expand as much, because your belly is pushing up on your diaphragm.

You also may have a condition called *sleep apnea,* which means that, when you sleep, you actually stop breathing for a period of time. You stop breathing because the tissues in your neck collapse in front of your windpipe, causing an obstruction when you're lying down. Sleep apnea can be mild to severe, and it needs to be identified and treated in certain individuals.

Your surgeon and your primary-care doctor will determine whether these conditions are significantly impairing your health and whether further testing can improve your particular lung condition.

Chest X-ray

A chest X-ray gives your doctor an image of your lungs that lets her know the general health of your lungs. A chest X-ray is required by most hospitals before you receive general anesthesia.

Chest CAT scan

If the results of the chest X-ray are abnormal, you'll need to have additional testing, including a chest CAT scan. The chest CAT scan gives more-detailed pictures of your lungs and the surrounding structures. You'll be hooked up to an IV and you'll probably be given an injection of a special dye that shows up on the CAT scan.

Oximetry

If you have severe asthma, sleep apnea, or a history of smoking, your doctor may send you to a *pulmonologist* (a doctor who specializes in the lungs). The pulmonologist may perform a number of tests, including an oximetry. In an oximetry, the doctor puts a clip on your finger that measures the percentage of oxygen in your blood.

Arterial blood gas

If you're sent to a pulmonologist, he will review the chest X-ray and also may get an *arterial blood gas,* in which blood is drawn with a needle out of the artery, usually from your wrist. Arteries carry oxygen from your lungs, so the arterial blood gas tells how well your lungs are getting oxygen into the blood and getting rid of one of the waste products, carbon dioxide. Not everyone needs to have the arterial blood gas done.

Spirometry

The pulmonologist also may put you through some pulmonary function tests, such as a spirometry. This test involves breathing into a tube with your nose plugged. The spirometry measures how well your lungs and airways move air. If you're severely obese or you suffer from asthma, your lungs may not expand as well as they should, and this test can help identify different problems with your breathing.

Sleep studies

Your surgeon may send you for a sleep study, looking for sleep apnea. If you have to undergo a sleep study, you'll likely have to go to a special center, known as a *sleep study center,* to have the test done. There, you'll be hooked up to some monitors to observe how you sleep. As you've probably guessed, the test usually is done at night.

The doctors are looking for any period of time when your breathing stops or when the percentage of oxygen in your blood drops below a normal level. These numbers are used to calculate what's known as a *sleep apnea index.* The sleep apnea index determines the severity of your sleep apnea and tells the doctors whether you require more testing for treatment. Treatment of sleep apnea requires another sleep study, where you wear a face mask that blows air out into your nose to keep those tissues from collapsing in front of your airway. This is known as *continuous positive airway pressure* (CPAP).

If a CPAP is prescribed for you, it's important that you use it. Some patients have difficulty with the equipment and don't use it for that reason. In this case, communicating with your physician to find something that works for you is important. Proper use of this mask really can help your breathing and blood-oxygen levels after surgery.

Gallbladder Tests

The gallbladder is attached to your liver and bile ducts and stores bile until the bile is needed to digest food. You can live without your gallbladder. In fact, surgery to remove the gallbladder is the most common surgical procedure done in the United States today.

Why all the fuss with gallbladders and weight loss surgery? As people lose weight rapidly (which is the goal after weight loss surgery), they can form gallstones, which can end up causing a blockage of one of the ducts draining the bile from the gallbladder. With this blockage comes a great deal of pain and inflammation of the gallbladder. This is a serious problem that requires removal of the gallbladder.

An ultrasound of your right upper abdomen can be done to determine whether you have gallstones. In most cases, the ultrasound will reveal stones if they're present.

Some surgeons always remove the gallbladder during weight loss surgery; other surgeons remove the gallbladder only in patients who've had a history of gallbladder attacks. Sometimes, however, even if you've had a history of gallbladder problems, your surgeon may not take out the gallbladder during the same operation. The decision of what to do with the gallbladder is really up to the surgeon — though you should definitely discuss it with your surgeon if you have a preference.

If you still have your gallbladder, in order to reduce stone formation, your surgeon may put you on the medication Actigall for several months after surgery.

Each surgery has its own risks. Weight loss surgery itself involves risks. And if you add other procedures — like gallbladder surgery — each of these procedures has its own, sometimes different, risks. Your surgeon should talk with you about the necessity of any surgeries in addition to your weight loss surgery.

Upper Gastrointestinal Tests

An upper gastrointestinal (GI) series looks at your esophagus, stomach, and some of your small intestine. You drink a liquid (barium or something equivalent), which doesn't taste very good. Then, using X-ray technology, your esophagus, stomach, and small intestine are outlined. This test helps your surgeon make sure that everything is as it should be. Specifically, the upper GI series usually can show the following:

- ✔ How well your esophagus functions

- ✔ Whether you have a *hiatal hernia* (where part of your stomach slips into the chest)

- ✔ In some cases, whether you have ulcers and growths in the stomach and intestines

Because it just shows an outline of your intestines, an upper GI series isn't as specific as an endoscopy, which actually shows your doctor how your insides look. Depending on several factors — including the type of surgery you're going to have, your medical history, and your surgeon's preference — you may need to have an upper endoscopy. You also may need to have an upper endoscopy if the upper GI series shows something like an ulcer or a growth.

In an upper endoscopy, a *gastroenterologist* (a doctor who specializes in the GI tract) or your surgeon will put a camera down your throat and take a look at your esophagus, stomach, and the first part of your small intestine, called the *duodenum*. (They try to make you comfortable during the procedure by giving you some medicine to numb your throat, as well as some IV drugs that make you just happy enough to tolerate the procedure without trying to strangle the doctor.) Your doctor is looking for any inflammation, ulcers, or growths that may need to be treated before your weight loss surgery. If you have an ulcer or severe inflammation, your surgery may be delayed until the ulcer or inflammation is treated and healed. In most cases, esophagitis or ulcers are treated for a minimum of 6 to 12 weeks — so don't put off this test until just before your surgery.

An *upper endoscopy* is technically called an *esophagogastroduodenoscopy,* or EGD — just in case you want to impress your doctor!

Colonoscopy

This test is not required before weight loss surgery unless you are 50 years old or older or have a strong family history of colon, breast, or ovarian cancer. In a colonoscopy, a doctor passes a tube up from your anus all the way around your colon (large intestine) to the point where your small intestine meets the colon. The tube has a lighted camera on the end and is about the width of your finger. A colonoscopy helps the doctor look for cancer, polyps, ulcers, pouches, and narrowed areas in your colon.

Colonoscopies are done because of medical history and family history. Regardless of whether you have a medical history or family history that requires a colonoscopy, if you're 50 years old, you'll likely need to have a colonoscopy, just to screen for cancer and other problems. The American Cancer Society recommends colonoscopies a minimum of once every ten years for everyone 50 and older.

Before the procedure, your doctor will give you instructions on how to "clean house." Normally you have to drink a gallon of liquid the evening before your test to clean out your colon. Colonoscopies are given under IV sedation, so you don't feel a thing.

Your surgeon doesn't touch your colon during weight loss surgery — it remains completely intact and unchanged. After you've had gastric bypass, you are *not* at increased risk when you need to have a colonoscopy.

Chapter 8

Preparing Yourself Physically and Mentally: Getting in Tip-Top Pre-Op Shape

*T*he better shape you're in going into your surgery, the better your chances of having a safe and successful experience. If your physical condition is very poor, the goal may be to maintain your weight and make sure your condition stays stable. But if you *can* improve your health, even slightly, prior to surgery, you'll be safer during the procedure.

In this chapter, we give you some tips on how you can improve your health before you enter the operating room. We also tell you about some of the ways you can prepare mentally and emotionally for your surgery.

Watching What You Eat Before Your Surgery

Many people who've made the decision to go through weight loss surgery think they'll never be able to eat again, and that leads them to binge before their surgery — eating far more than they would normally, all in an effort to have their "last supper" (even if it's for weeks on end). The *last supper syndrome* is the behavior of many patients as they try to eat their way to the operating room. As a result, many gain weight just prior to surgery.

The truth is, after you reach your weight loss goal, you'll probably be able to enjoy a bite or two of foods you thought you would never eat again. Many patients find that their pouches give them the control they need to be completely satisfied by just a small taste.

Gaining additional weight just before surgery only adds to obesity-related health problems. Here are some dangers to consider:

- **If you're suffering from respiratory problems from having too much tissue in the area of your throat, additional weight gain will only add to that tissue and cause more respiratory difficulty.**

- **As you gain more weight, more fat may be deposited into your liver, and your liver may become larger.** The liver is located close to where your surgeon will be operating. Gaining additional weight can increase the size of your liver, so it can be in the path of surgery. If this happens, you may be at a higher risk having your surgery performed as an open procedure rather than a laparoscopic procedure or not having the procedure at all. Losing weight can help to shrink the liver so it's less vulnerable.

- **The more weight you gain, the more stress is put on your heart as your heart works harder to pump oxygen to all parts of your body.** Any major surgery will stress the heart. Additional weight will increase that stress.

Remember: Treating every meal before surgery as if it were your last isn't worth the risk.

Although it's true that, in the first few months, the quantity of food you'll be able to consume will be very limited (because your new stomach will be swollen), you'll eventually be able to eat larger quantities. You never want to return to the days when you could eat huge amounts (after all, that's what got you to the point of needing weight loss surgery in the first place), but your new stomach will probably expand slightly, and in gastric bypass, the opening out of your pouch into your intestines can expand. A year or two after surgery, you'll probably long for those days when you could just nibble and feel completely full.

Some surgeons require that their patients lose weight prior to surgery. Here's why:

- ✔ **Successful weight loss surgery requires that the patient be committed to a healthier lifestyle.** The surgeon wants to ensure that you can make that commitment by losing a certain amount of weight prior to surgery.

- ✔ **Losing weight will cause the liver to shrink in those who have a fatty liver.** This will, in turn, make your surgery safer. Some surgeons put you on a two-week high-protein, liquid diet to get your liver smaller.

- ✔ **Even if you don't lose weight, at least you're far less likely to gain a lot of weight prior to surgery if you're following a diet.**

Doing Exercises to Improve Your Fitness

To be in the best shape possible before surgery, start your exercise program now. Wait, wait . . . don't throw this book across the room! We don't mean that you need to join a gym, buy a Speedo, hire a personal trainer, and achieve instant fitness. We mean you should just start moving, regardless of your ability. Do what you can for as long as you can, and try to do it every day.

The following sections give you some tips for physical exercises and breathing exercises that can improve your fitness before your surgery.

ANECDOTE

You can eat after surgery

I thought when I had weight loss surgery that I would never be able to eat again. For some reason I thought that, for the rest of my life, I'd survive on a few bites of food several times a day and be done or full. Boy, was I wrong! About six months after surgery, I realized that I was able to eat more than those "few bites" and that I had to be responsible for everything I put in my mouth. I can't eat like I could before my surgery, but I can eat like a "normal" person—not a 300-pound person, but a 160-pound person. I have to be conscious of portions, sugars, and fats, but I can still eat! Having weight loss surgery doesn't mean you're going to starve or not be able to go out to dinner with family and friends. It just means you may need a takeout box! It's all about moderation and being responsible, the hardest thing I've ever had to do in my life.

Jackie Hutchison
Newport, Michigan

Physical exercises

Every little bit of exercise helps when you're facing weight loss surgery — whether it's walking, doing water aerobics, or exercising along with a TV show, video, or DVD. You aren't necessarily expected to be able to start a rigorous fitness program now if your doctor and your physical condition dictate otherwise — but try to move as much as you can, under the advice of your doctor. You'll be healthier and safer for the effort.

Try one or both of the following:

- ✔ **Walking:** Walk around the neighborhood and count houses. See how many houses you can walk past and, by the time of your surgery, try to increase that number. If you live near a shopping mall, strolling through the mall can be a fun activity, especially in the winter when you can't always walk outdoors.

- ✔ **Swimming or water fitness:** If swimming isn't your thing, you can get in the water and march in place, do squats, or walk from one side of the shallow end of the pool to the other side of the shallow end.

Here are some signs to watch out for. If you experience any of the following symptoms, you know it's time to stop exercising and consult a doctor immediately:

- ✔ Dizziness or nausea
- ✔ Chest, neck, or arm pain
- ✔ Difficulty breathing or gasping for air

Now is also a great time to plan for the exercise program you'll follow after your surgery. If you plan ahead, you're more likely to start right in rather than procrastinating. Turn to Chapter 16 for more on physical fitness.

Breathing exercises

Practicing breathing exercises prior to surgery can have a very beneficial effect. It helps to improve your heart function, exercises your lungs, and reduces stress.

You know you're breathing properly if your stomach moves when you're breathing. Start by inhaling deeply so that it feels as though you're filling your lower lungs with air. Place your hands lightly on your stomach and concentrate on making your hands move up.

WARNING!

Butting out: No smoking!

Smoking is a harmful activity even if you aren't about to undergo weight loss surgery, but it's especially harmful for weight loss surgery patients. If you smoke, you absolutely *must* stop smoking at *least* four to eight weeks before surgery. Smoking prevents the proper functioning of your lungs, as well as adds stress to your heart. Many surgeons won't operate on patients who aren't able to stop smoking. Here's why:

✔ If you can't quit smoking, some surgeons reason that you won't have the commitment to go through all the life changes that will be required of you after weight loss surgery.

✔ Severe obesity and problems with breathing go hand in hand. If you smoke, your ability to breathe is made worse. Your lungs won't be clear of phlegm, and breathing after surgery is jeopardized. You may have difficulty waking up from anesthesia, and you're at an increased risk of pneumonia.

✔ Weight loss surgery is a very serious procedure requiring a lot of healing. Healing takes place when the blood supply brings oxygen to the affected area. Smoking decreases the oxygen in the blood supply because, instead of inhaling air, you're inhaling cigarette smoke.

✔ Nicotine in cigarette smoke is an irritant. The main cause of stomach ulcers in newly formed pouches following surgery is smoking.

For information on how to quit, visit the American Cancer Society website at www.cancer.org or the American Lung Association at www.lung usa.org.

If that wasn't enough to convince you to stop smoking, consider this: The American Society of Anesthesiologists presented a study of 500 patients undergoing outpatient surgery. Those patients who smoked within 24 hours of having general anesthesia were found to be 20 times more likely to have inadequate oxygen supply to the heart during surgery.

You also may want to start coughing exercises. This is something you'll need to do when you're in the hospital to clear your lungs. Breathe deeply, filling your lower lungs and, as you exhale, cough twice. Do this four or five times per day. It will help clear your lungs of phlegm and open up the air sacs in the lungs.

Try this breathing exercise every day until your surgery:

1. **Lie on the floor with your knees bent, your head on a pillow, and your hands on your stomach.**

   If lying on the floor is too uncomfortable, do the exercise sitting in a chair.

2. **Breathe in over a count of four so you feel like your lower lungs are full and you can feel your stomach rise.**

3. **Hold your breath for a count of four, and slowly exhale for a count of four.**

   Repeat that four more times.

4. **Lie or sit comfortably for a minute relaxing.**

   You'll feel rejuvenated.

   Over the course of a few days, work your way up to holding your breath for a slow count of four, and slowly exhale. Then try a slow count of five.

Getting Organized

Getting yourself organized for your return home from the hospital will pay off in many ways. You'll be better able to concentrate on yourself and your new way of life. Some patients are better able to handle the surgery and bounce back readily, while others report that they feel as though they were hit by a truck. To be on the safe side, be ready for anything.

Stocking your kitchen

Although you won't be able to eat and drink very much after surgery, you'll need to have some specific things on hand for your return home. Here are some good choices for that first week or two:

- **Canned broth:** Select from chicken, beef, or vegetable. Four cans should be more than enough — you'll be consuming only ¼ cup at a time.

- **Diet Jell-O:** You can have any flavor, any time.

- **Sugar-free popsicles:** These are wonderfully refreshing, and because you have to eat them slowly, they help teach you to eat slowly.

- **Pureed soup like butternut squash**

- **Low-fat, no-sugar-added yogurt**

- **Sugar-free pudding:** Try adding unflavored protein powder to make it more nutritious.

Try to choose foods and drinks you think you'll enjoy.

Let it snow, let it snow, let it snow . . .

My lifesaver post-op was a little snow-cone machine. The first two weeks at home were very hard. I couldn't drink much of anything, and everything seemed to upset my stomach. I could tolerate ice well in the hospital, so my daughter brought home a snow-cone machine for me to try. It worked wonders. I added a little juice to it for flavor.

Janet Santos
Tiverton, Rhode Island

Preparing your home

Be sure that your home environment is ready for your return from the hospital. You may want special equipment or furniture. The following may make your post-op life a little easier:

- ✓ **Hospital bed:** If you place it on the same floor as your kitchen and bathroom, it may be a relief during the first week or two following surgery. Check with your insurance carrier regarding how this may be arranged if it seems like it will be a necessity. The social-service department of your hospital also can help with this.

- ✓ **Reclining chair:** If you have one, you may end up sleeping in it if you're too uncomfortable to sleep in bed immediately following your surgery. Sometimes patients feel a tugging or pulling on the stitches in their abdominal area when lying flat in bed. It's important to keep your legs elevated. Wherever you rest best is the place to sleep.

- ✓ **Shower chair:** Many weight loss surgery patients have these going into surgery, but if you don't, consider getting one. You'll be unsteady following your surgery because of the anesthesia, rapid weight loss, and possible associated low blood pressure. A shower chair will provide you with an important measure of safety.

You also want to be sure you have a thermometer, liquid Tylenol, and a blender for mixing protein supplements. A pill cutter or crusher is also good to have. Check with your pharmacist or doctor if your medications can be opened or crushed.

Tying up the loose ends

Weight loss surgery is serious surgery that requires you to take it easy when you get home. You'll want to be able to concentrate on healing and not be faced with life's little annoyances. Taking care of loose ends ahead of time will give you the freedom to do that.

Here are some details to take care of before you go to the hospital:

✔ **Pay all outstanding bills (and, if you can, try paying ahead).** If your surgery doesn't go as smoothly as you hope it will and you end up having to stay in the hospital far longer than expected, your bills will be taken care of.

✔ **Have your prescriptions filled, especially your pain medications.** Nothing is worse than leaving the hospital in pain and having to stop at the pharmacy for pain relief.

✔ **Return all library books and rented movies.** You don't want to be taking care of small errands immediately after your surgery.

✔ **Clean your house and do your laundry.** Don't count on being able to do either of these chores right after your return home. (If a less-than-sparkling house and some dirty laundry won't bother you, don't worry about doing it beforehand.)

✔ **Stock up on magazines and short stories.** Don't expect to be able to read serious novels right after your surgery. The aftereffects of anesthesia will make concentrating more difficult. Magazines and short stories are far better.

Bowel prep: You've got to be kidding

If you're having the Roux-en-Y gastric bypass surgery or the duodenal switch, your surgery will involve your intestines. Some surgeons require a bowel prep before surgery so the intestines are free of, well, you get the idea.

Your surgeon will give you specific instructions, but here's what you can generally expect: You'll need to drink clear liquids such as clear broth, ginger ale, and Jell-O on the day before surgery. You'll also either use a commercial enema or laxative product such as Fleet Phospho-Soda, GoLYTELY, Dulcolax, or Miralax.

Don't plan any activities during that time. You will need to be close to a bathroom and will probably be quite uncomfortable. Plan to do nothing but relax.

Psyching Yourself Up for Surgery

Weight loss surgery is not the easy way out. It's a tool that will help you to find health and a more normal way of life. However, you play the greatest role in this process. Your own mental attitude and commitment to success will lead to your success or failure following surgery.

Going through weight loss surgery takes a tremendous amount of courage. You may have some worries and fears going into the surgery. Do everything you can to talk with your surgeon, the psychologist, and other weight loss surgery patients about what you can expect. The fewer lingering questions you have when you leave home for the hospital, the better you'll be able to focus on your number-one priority: recuperating well.

In the following sections, we help you do some mental and emotional work to get yourself ready for the journey ahead.

Taking stock of where you are going into the surgery

Are you one to dive for cover when the camera comes out? Most patients have very few pictures of themselves, because they don't want a permanent reminder of how they look. That time is over. Swallow your pride and have those pictures taken from all sides and all angles, in all outfits, including shorts and even bathing suits. These pictures will become a symbol of an important starting point for a wonderful journey.

Take the time to fill out the worksheet in this chapter, as a record of your starting point. Here's why the record of your starting point is important:

- You'll undoubtedly hit a plateau at some point in your post-op journey. At those times, you won't be losing weight, but you may be losing inches. Your record of your measurements will verify that you're still changing, regardless of what the scale says.

- If at any time you don't feel like you've done as well as you would have liked, look at those before pictures for an affirmation of your success. People have a tendency to forget how really bad things were prior to surgery.

- A year or two after your surgery, people will swear they never knew you when you were really that heavy. Take out your before pictures and jog their memory. They'll have a renewed appreciation for your determination.

- Many patients keep a record of their weight loss progress through pictures and measurements and make a scrapbook of their journey. It can be something you treasure and proudly display. Having a scrapbook without that beginning picture, weight, and measurements would be a shame.

My Starting Point

Date: _____

Weight: _____

Bust Measurement: _____

Waist Measurement: _____

Hip Measurement: _____

Upper-Arm Measurement: _____

Thigh Measurement: _____

Neck Measurement: _____

Attach your before picture here

Illustration by Wiley, Composition Services Graphics

My journal experience

Something that was very important to me was mental preparation. It helped me to know what to expect and to realize that I was going to learn much more.

I started my journal-writing experience 30 days prior to surgery with the focus on making my goals important by writing them down. I knew that if times got tough, I would remember why I was doing this and reflect back and remember my goals. I also wanted to celebrate my achievements, and not lose sight of their importance to my journey.

I hadn't been a journal or diary writer in the past, so this was a new experience for me. I now relish reading back in my journal and re-experiencing the lessons I learned in the first few months with my new tummy. This was the difference between my weight loss surgery and all the other diets that I had been on and failed in

the past. I took every new step as a sign of what was good for my body, whether it was water, water, and more water; having protein first; avoiding refined carbohydrates; or eating slowly and chewing thoroughly.

For the first month or two, my goal was to write every day, and there was always something to jot down. Now my goal is every week, which tends to act as a reinforcement. I record all the successes of being a smaller size. I record all the positives of feeling fit, running up the stairs and not being winded, and wearing form-fitting clothes that don't have to camouflage my shape. I still have another 30 to 40 pounds to go in order to reach my goal, and I know that I can achieve it.

Susan Hartmann
East Windsor, New Jersey

Journaling

Start a journal or diary before your surgery and keep it up afterward. It'll be a reminder of your thoughts and experiences along the way. You may want to blog about your experiences — try Blogger (www.blogger.com) or Tumblr (www.tumblr.com) — or tweet about them (www.twitter.com). You also can share your experiences on the Facebook page WLS Private, hosted by author Barbara Thompson; you can find this private group by joining Facebook (www.facebook.com) and searching for "WLS Private."

After surgery, you'll struggle with food or hit plateaus, and you'll need a reminder of just how difficult life was prior to surgery. Your words will remind you of how it felt to be severely obese, how your health problems plagued you, and how much your life has changed for the better.

By keeping a record of your food intake, your moods, your exercise, and how much water you drink, you can compare what worked for you and what didn't. If your weight is slowing or at a standstill, you'll be able to make a comparison to when you were losing weight. This will help you to determine if you're straying or if your body is just going through a temporary plateau. Record your weight and your measurements, as well as your clothing sizes.

Weight loss surgery is about more than losing weight. It's about achieving a healthier, more satisfying way of life. Going into your surgery, you can probably list many things that you'd love to do if you were of normal weight. By recording those things, they become tangible goals that you'll have a far greater chance of achieving because you've written them down. Sometimes, your goals or targets change. When you see what your goals were, it gives you a sense of accomplishment because of what you've achieved and can fuel you to a greater success!

Part III

The Hospital Experience and Beyond

The 5th Wave   By Rich Tennant

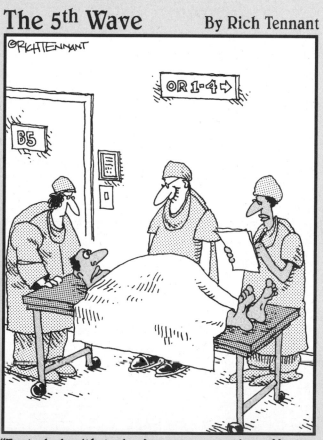

"Included with today's surgery, we're offering a manicure, pedicure, haircut, and ear wax flush for just $49.95."

In this part . . .

What will your time in the hospital be like? In this part, we tell you all about the tests, strategies, and procedures that you can expect while you're there. We also tell you how to eat and what to eat from those first days through the first few months. In this part, you find recipes and menus to help you on your way.

Family and friends play an important role while you're in the hospital and provide much-needed support at home. And when you're ready to go back to work, we help you handle questions from co-workers.

Chapter 9

Checking In and Out: Your Hospital Stay

. . . .

In This Chapter

▶ Gathering the support you need

▶ Getting moving while you're in the hospital

▶ Looking out for your comfort

▶ Getting to go home

. . . .

*Y*ou've decided to have the surgery, you've set the date, you've packed your bags, and now it's time to leave for the hospital. It's only natural to feel some nervousness and anxiety, because you're not quite sure what to expect.

In this chapter, we try to allay your concerns by telling you exactly what to expect while you're in the hospital. We also show you how you can make your stay more comfortable and what you can do while you're in the hospital to speed up your recovery. Finally, we take a look at your trip home and show you how to make it as easy as possible.

Knowing What Affects the Length of Your Stay

No one wants to stay in the hospital, and everyone wants to get back to the comforts of home as soon as possible. So, how long will you have to be in the hospital? The length of your stay will depend upon many different factors. In the following sections, we cover several of the major ones.

Try not to be in too big a hurry to return home. You'll certainly be more comfortable there, but you've just had major surgery, and your surgeon is the best judge of when discharging you is safe. Being severely obese brings its own set of problems regarding surgery. Your breathing must be clear, your heart must be stable, you shouldn't have a fever, and you should be able to drink liquids and do some things for yourself before you leave the hospital. You need to be able to get to the bathroom by yourself, get yourself something to drink and eat, shower, get out of bed by yourself, and dress yourself.

Type of surgery

The length of your hospital stay depends upon the type of surgery you've had and whether your surgery was done as an open incision or laparoscopically. With gastric banding surgery, the hospital stay is normally one day. Gastric bypass, sleeve gastrectomy, and duodenal switch surgeries done laparoscopically require about a two- to three-day stay. Procedures done with an open incision require about a four- to six-day stay.

Your physical condition

The length of your stay will certainly depend upon your own physical condition. If you have illnesses that put you at an increased risk, you may have to stay a little longer. This is especially true if you have a serious heart condition or severe respiratory problems.

You'll also remain in the hospital longer if you have a fever. Your surgeon will want to find the cause of the fever and treat it before sending you home.

Support at home

The length of your hospital stay also may depend upon how much support you have at home. If you have great support from someone who can be very attentive to your needs, your surgeon may be more inclined to discharge you earlier.

When you're home with all this great support and help, don't make the mistake of lying around. You need to walk to get your blood flowing in your legs so you prevent blood clots from forming. So, walk, then rest, then repeat the cycle.

You'll be drinking and in some cases having pureed food when you return home, so food preparation is not a major issue, but your ability to do anything for the rest of your family will be very limited. Expect to feel fatigued for up to six to eight weeks after surgery. You'll probably be able to go to work, and do the things you have to at home after two to three weeks, but be prepared to go to bed early!

Travel

If you've traveled a distance to have your surgery, you'll most likely be discharged to stay in a hotel near the hospital. Many surgeons make arrangements with hotels for out-of-town patients so you receive favorable rates. Room service even may provide you with a clear liquid diet during your stay. Or the arrangements may be with a suite hotel, so you can have your own food in your room. Generally, you'll stay in the hotel for a week to ten days until you've met with your surgeon for the follow-up appointment and been cleared to travel.

If at all possible, have someone stay with you in the hotel. Going through this experience alone can be very lonely and possibly depressing — you'll need some company during this time. If you don't know anyone who can stay with you, ask the surgeon if he can recommend a former patient who lives locally who may be able to spend some time with you. You'd be surprised at the network of people who will volunteer to come to your aid — people who've gone through what you're going through and will understand.

While you're in the hotel, be sure to walk the hallways. Staying in a room for an extended period of time won't help your recovery. You need to get out and move. Most hotels have a fitness room with a treadmill. Ask your surgeon if you can start slowly using the treadmill.

The Company You Keep: Having Family with You

Having family members or close friends stay with you while you're in the hospital can be very comforting. They're there to help you get in and out of bed, get whatever you may need, and commiserate with you. A family member or friend will respond immediately if you need anything, whereas a nurse may not have the freedom of time to help you right away with non-life-threatening requests.

Getting a patient advocate to work on your behalf

A patient advocate is employed by the hospital to be a liaison between the patient and the hospital staff. This person helps you to understand hospital policy and obtain any services that you need. She's there to ensure you get the care you need when you need it. She'll only intervene on your behalf if you call her and ask for her assistance. The services of a patient advocate are free. When in the hospital, just ask the hospital operator to connect you with the patient advocate. Patient advocates can be an invaluable asset.

Here are some things your family member or friend can do:

- Feed you ice chips and make sure you have an adequate supply of mouth swabs
- Help put your compression leggings on or take them off
- Help take you to the bathroom
- Walk the halls with you, making sure not only that you do it but that you don't trip on your IVs
- Request any medication you may need
- Keep you company
- Adjust the bed up or down
- Get washcloths for your face
- Alert the nursing staff when medication refills are needed
- Tuck in your covers
- Make sure you use your *spirometer* (a simple breathing device given to you in the hospital to help clear your lungs)

Your family and friends also will be there to speak up for you if you feel your treatment is less than ideal. Family and friends shouldn't be on the lookout for things to complain about, of course — hospital staff members are very often overworked and underappreciated. But if there is a serious problem with your treatment, your family and friends may be able to speak for you when you can't speak for yourself.

Having your family and friends in the hospital also involves them in your weight loss surgery journey right from the beginning. The more your family and friends feel part of what you're going through, the more understanding and supportive they're likely to be. Going through the surgery with you will make your significant other feel closer to you during this life-altering experience.

In some cases, your family and friends will be able to stay in your room the entire time if space permits and if you have a private room. In other cases, they'll only be permitted during visiting hours. The wing where you'll be staying may be used primarily for weight loss surgery patients; you may have a private room. The bariatric coordinator will know if family members routinely stay with patients. If a private room is not guaranteed, call the hospital and see what arrangements you can make if this is something that's important to you.

You love them, but you may have family members or friends who would be more trouble than help if they stayed with you at the hospital. Whether they're not accustomed to helping out, they complain constantly, or they're just not supportive of you and your decision to have surgery, you don't need them around. When you aren't feeling well or you're trying to heal, you need a more positive environment. Better to say thanks but no thanks if they volunteer to stay with you.

You also may not want a lot of visitors when you're in the hospital. Even if you aren't in a lot of pain, you'll feel like you were hit by a truck. Comfort and solace may be appreciated, but at least for your first day, suggest that people stay away.

My soul mate

I have been married for over 29 years to the same man. When I decided to have weight loss surgery, his first reaction was somewhat negative. But he attended the support-group meeting and the bari boot camp with me, where he met my surgeon and his staff. He was won over.

He went with me to the hospital and did not come home until I did. We spent two nights and three days in the hospital. He slept in a chair at my bedside and encouraged me to take ice chips, breathe deeply, and move my legs. When

I was able to get up, he helped me walk the halls. I so appreciated him and his support.

I am now 108 pounds lighter, off my blood pressure medication (which I had taken for 20 years), off my CPAP and feel better than I ever would have dreamed. My surgery not only saved my life, it gave me a better quality of life. Our personal relationship — which has always been very good — is closer than ever. He is my soul mate.

Sandy Fields
East Bernstadt, Kentucky

"Aide"ing Your Recovery: Nurses and Other Staff

Your nurse is your advocate and the first in line to identify problems. Most hospitals that do a lot of bariatric surgery have designated hospital wards and, therefore, designated nurses who take care of weight loss surgery patients. They're familiar with how you should look after surgery and can usually identify when something is wrong. They do, however, follow a specific care plan, so if you require more care or don't fit into the standard care plan, you may be moved to a different floor.

Your nurse will come in to check on you throughout the day. Nurses work in shifts that can be 8 to 12 hours long. ***Remember:*** Your nurse is taking care of several patients at one time. Plus, your nurse has to document everything that has happened with each patient during the course of the day. Your nurse's day is probably very busy, which usually means you don't see your nurse every second of the day. Your nurse will have an aide who helps her get all the work done.

Your nurse and your nurse's aide are your advocates. They're on your side even if they can't always be *at* your side.

You can expect to see another staff member who draws your blood or puts in IV catheters. If you need to have an X-ray done, another staff member will bring you back and forth from the test. When you go to the radiology department for X-rays, be prepared for the possibility that you may be down there for a while. The people who bring you to radiology will leave you to take other people back to their rooms, so you may have to wait around. It can be a little cold in radiology. If you've been using pain medication, ask your nurse to give you something before you go to radiology so you'll be more comfortable.

If you're in a teaching hospital

Some hospitals train doctors who have just graduated from medical school in different fields of medicine — these recent graduates are known as *residents.* The training programs, called *residencies,* can be anywhere from three to six years in duration. You may be worrying that you're serving as a guinea pig for residents, but this isn't actually the case. Residents are supervised by doctors who've completed their training and been in practice for years.

Having residents in a hospital is a good thing because, invariably, in the middle of the night or at odd times during the day, there is always a doctor around who can help you. The residents will contact your doctor for you if there is a serious problem, and they can start treatment in the meantime.

The hospital's dietitian will go over what, how, and when you should eat when you go home. Pay careful attention, read through the materials you get, and ask the dietitian to come back if you have any more questions. The most important things you'll hear is chew, chew, chew; don't eat and drink at the same time; and avoid using straws. Practice this in the hospital. If you go home on a liquid diet, pay attention anyway. Your time in the sun is just a few days away, and forewarned is forearmed.

A *nutritionist* is someone who has taken some classes in nutrition. A *dietitian* has studied nutrition extensively and is registered and licensed by the state.

Making Your Stay More Comfortable

Even though your first days in the hospital won't be very pleasant, you can make some preparations and follow some techniques that will lessen your pain or discomfort. We cover these in the following sections.

Knowing what to bring to the hospital

Here's a list of items that weight loss surgery patients have found extremely helpful during their hospital stay:

- **Pillow:** Not only will you rest better if you have your own pillow, but you'll be able to use it to help you move. You'll also have it for the ride home.

- **Your journal:** Keep a record of your hospital experience. You'll be so happy when you've reached your goal weight to be able to go back over your hospital stay and remember what you went through, as well as appreciate how far you've come.

- **Loose-fitting clothes for the trip home.**

- **Small fan:** Many patients have appreciated having a fan to stay cool. If you do bring a fan, be prepared to give it to the hospital maintenance or engineering department first to have them make sure it's safe to be used in the hospital and up to their code requirements. Your family members can do this for you while they're waiting for you during your surgery.

- **CPAP machine:** If you use one to help you breathe because of sleep apnea, check with your surgeon about this prior to surgery. Some surgeons want you to bring your own machine; others do not.

- **Lip balm:** This is great for dry lips, which are common after surgery.

- ✔ **Talcum powder:** This is good for overall comfort.

- ✔ **Pictures of those you love:** They'll remind you that you're having this surgery not only for yourself, but so you can be around a lot longer with the people you love.

- ✔ **Camera:** Many patients take great pride and pleasure in keeping a complete record of all their experiences, and this record includes pictures. If you're interested in keeping this kind of record, have someone take pictures of you while you're in the hospital.

- ✔ **Toiletry items.**

- ✔ **Insurance card.**

- ✔ **Slippers:** Make sure they have no-skid soles to prevent falls on slippery hospital floors. Also, choose slippers you can put on easily without bending.

- ✔ **Medications you've been taking and that your surgeon says it's okay for you to continue taking:** Any medications you've been taking at home have to be cleared by your surgeon before you can continue taking them. If you bring your medication from home to the hospital, don't take it unless specifically instructed by your surgeon. And make sure to let your nurse know.

- ✔ **This book!**

Getting out of bed

If you don't have a special bariatric bed that folds into a chair shape so you can step out of bed, you'll have to use your abdominal muscles to help you. Because this can be somewhat painful, here's a technique that will help:

1. **Turn over on your right side and cross your left arm over in front of you.**

2. **Use your left arm to push yourself up so you can swing your legs down.**

3. **As you start to lift, use your right arm to push yourself up into a sitting position.**

   You can reverse everything when you need to roll over on your left side to get out of bed.

Many bariatric beds also have a triangular-shaped trapeze over the bed. If you raise the head of your bed so you're in more of a sitting position, you can grab this triangle to lift yourself up as you swing your legs around.

TECHNICAL STUFF

Tubes, glorious tubes

You'll encounter a variety of tubes during your hospital stay. The tubes you have will vary depending upon the preference of your doctor and your own physical condition. If you're interested, check with your surgeon to find out exactly which tubes you'll have. But here is a list of some you may encounter:

✔ **Breathing tube:** This tube will be placed down your throat during surgery to help you breathe. It's put in just before surgery and usually removed after surgery. (You probably won't have any memory of when the tube is put in or removed, because you'll be going under or coming out of anesthesia.) The tube ensures that you have a clear passage for air to go to the lungs. The tube is attached to a respirator to aid your breathing during surgery and sometimes after the surgery until you're completely able to breathe on your own.

✔ **Urinary catheter:** This is a tube that is inserted into your urethra so that your urine is collected in a bag. This is normally done in the operating room when you're under general anesthesia, so you have no idea it's happening. The thought of this may be unpleasant, but after surgery, if you're in a lot of pain, not having to worry about getting up to go to the bathroom is nice. The catheter will stay in a day or two depending upon your mobility and your overall health.

✔ **Drainage tubes:** Some surgeons will insert a drainage tube into the abdominal area called a Jackson-Pratt (JP) drain. This tube comes out of the body, attaches to a plastic bottle, and drains fluid from inside your belly. In some cases, after open surgery, the drain is placed in the abdominal wall to prevent the collection of fluids. The bottle looks a little like a soft hand grenade. The bottle is squeezed, and it works to suction the fluid out of the area. When the bottle is about half-full, it needs to be emptied.

If the bottle gets too full, it can't create the proper suction to remove the fluids from your body. If there is any infection in the abdominal area, it gets the fluid out of the body and keeps you healthy.

Some surgeons remove the JP drain before you leave the hospital. Others have you go home with it. When you leave the hospital with the JP drain in place, you'll need to collect and measure the fluid and report the amount to your surgeon at your next visit. You'll also need to make note of the color of the fluid and any odor. The fluid should be clear, have a slight pink tinge to it, and have no odor. If the fluid is milky and/or has a bad odor, you need to report this to your doctor right away; this is a sign of infection.

The JP drain may stay in for up to ten days. When you go to see your surgeon at your first checkup, the tube will normally be removed in the office by the nurse. To remove the tube, it's just pulled out. Hold your breath while it's being taken out — it's over in about 3 seconds. When the drain is in, it's covered by a gauze bandage. When removed, the very small opening doesn't have to be stitched — it's just covered by gauze and will heal on its own.

Most patients are happy to be free of the JP drain. It can get in the way when you wear clothes. Having it removed also makes you feel like you're on your way to recovery and healing just fine.

✔ **Nasogastric tube:** In some cases, you may need a tube in your nose called a *nasogastric tube.* This tube is rarely used after laparoscopic surgery; it's more frequently used after open surgery. Ask your surgeon ahead of time whether you'll have one of these, so you know what to expect.

Getting the right pillow

The pillow can be one of your best friends while you're in the hospital, especially if it's your own pillow. It will help you to rest better and also can be a comfort and an aid when you're moving. Clutch your pillow to your abdomen and hold it firmly against your stomach. This will give support for your abdomen and will help with the pain.

Specially designed pillows are available just for this purpose. Some are shaped like teddy bears but have a hard back for added support. They combine the psychological comfort of a bear and the therapeutic support of a pillow. They're also great to hold when you cough. ***Remember:*** You have to get that air moving and open up all the air pockets in your lungs.

The occupational therapist can help with these and other techniques (see "Taking advantage of physical therapy," later in this chapter).

Wearing compression stockings

You'll be given some type of compression stockings to wear during your hospital stay. These will help reduce the risk of deep venous thrombosis (DVT), which are the blood clots that can form in a patient's legs after surgery. These blood clots can lead to pulmonary embolism, which is a very serious condition (see Chapter 4).

Compression stockings are about twice the thickness of regular stockings, fit very tightly over the calf of the leg up to the knee, and are very difficult to put on.

Most hospitals provide leg devices that are more effective and sophisticated than compression stockings. These look more like leggings. When you put them on, air is pumped into them and pumped out so there is a squeezing or kneading massage action on your legs.

Using a bariatric bed and equipment

Hospitals use a variety of types of beds and equipment. Before your surgery, ask the bariatric coordinator at your surgeon's office about how the hospital is equipped.

Many patients are embarrassed that they need special accommodations during their stay. However, for this surgery, you just have to swallow your pride. You can reasonably expect that if bariatric surgery is performed at a hospital, the hospital should be able to accommodate your size. Centers of Excellence (see Chapter 5) are required to have the appropriate equipment.

This equipment is not only a comfort concern but a safety concern. Most hospitals do a good job in having the right size equipment, but with so much demand, there may be a shortage.

You may want to contact the patient advocate if the size of your bed or the equipment is not appropriate. If your safety and comfort are an issue, don't be shy about speaking up.

Bariatric beds

Bariatric beds are designed for patients who weigh more than 350 pounds. If your weight going into the surgery is more than 350 pounds, you shouldn't be in a regular-size bed. It will be too small and uncomfortable for you and may not bear your weight; plus, you'll have a harder time getting out of bed.

Some bariatric beds fold so when you're ready to get out of bed, the bed will look like a chair, and all you have to do is stand up. Bariatric beds also have special pressure-relief air mattresses so you're less likely to get pressure ulcers when you're lying in bed. They're also much wider than traditional beds and have heavy-duty handrails.

Wheelchairs

The hospital should have an adequate supply of large wheelchairs. Some large wheelchairs accommodate up to only 350 pounds. If you weigh more than 350 pounds, check the weight limit of the wheelchairs at the hospital. If during your stay, you're asked to get into a wheelchair that doesn't fit you, you have every right (legally speaking) to refuse the chair and request a larger one.

Bathroom accommodations

If your weight exceeds 350 pounds, your bathroom should be equipped with a commode that is mounted to the floor rather than to the wall. You may have an extra-wide shower, although not all hospitals are equipped with these.

You also may have a bedside commode that is wider, can support weight in excess of your own weight, and has side bars that come down.

Gowns

Your hospital should absolutely have a gown that fits you appropriately. If for some reason the hospital doesn't have gowns in your size, you can wear two gowns — one with the opening in the front and another with the opening in the back — though it'll be quite warm.

You can wear your own gown if you prefer, but be sure that whatever you wear has short sleeves. You'll have IVs in your arm, so you won't be able to wear long sleeves.

Taking pain medication

Your surgeons will discuss with you measures for reducing your pain. A variety of pain medications and methods of delivering them are available. What you're given will probably be based upon the experience your surgeon has had with other patients. If you've had previous surgeries, you may know what you prefer; if so, be sure to discuss that with your doctor before your surgery.

In most cases, you'll have a narcotic delivered intravenously, and you'll control the dosage with a *patient-controlled analgesia* (PCA). This machine is designed to allow you to give yourself more medicine when you feel you need it, without allowing you to inadvertently overmedicate yourself. The doctor or nurse will set it up so you can press a button to give yourself a dose of medication through your intravenous tube when you feel the need. But the settings will allow only a maximum number of doses within a certain time span.

If you have difficulty with your pain medication, have the nurse report this to your surgeon so adjustments can be made. If the pain medication doesn't agree with you, you can request that it be changed. Many pain medications are available, and your doctor can order another one if you're feeling nausea.

Your pain medication also may not be strong enough. The medication dosage is based upon the average amount of medicine based upon your particular weight. If you're still feeling pain, the dosage can be increased or another type of medication can be tried.

Have discussions about pain medication with your surgeon prior to surgery so she can note contingency plans on your hospital record. Nurses will generally wait until the doctor is in the hospital visiting patients to bring up problems such as pain medication. It may be hours before your surgeon is back in the hospital on rounds, and you may be in a lot of pain all that time. Have this addressed early, especially if you've had problems with pain medication in the past.

Doing Everything You Can to Speed Up Your Recovery

You can do a lot to make your recovery smoother and faster. In the following sections, we give you some concrete suggestions.

Walk this way: Exercise starts in the hospital

You'll be expected to walk the same day as your surgery. Although you may complain bitterly about this, getting up and walking really is quite important. You may be able to take only a few steps that first day, but the more you can move, the better off you'll be.

Walking will be made a bit more difficult because you'll be carting along the IV fluid and machine on a pole, a urinary bag, and possibly drains. Have a walking companion — a family member, a friend, or a nurse. That person can help you cope with all the tubes.

By the time you leave the hospital, you should be walking the halls. Just be sure to continue this walking program when you get home. Of course, you'll only be asked to walk if your vital signs are good and you're feeling as well as can be expected for having had major surgery.

Walking after your surgery is important for a number of reasons:

- It officially starts your exercise program from day one.
- It helps in the healing process.
- It helps you to pass gas.
- It helps your lungs to open up.
- It helps to guard against blood clots.
- It helps you feel better overall.

Every breath you take: Using your spirometer

With inactivity in the hospital, the small air sacs or pockets in your lungs may start to close or to collect fluid. When the air sacs close, this is called *atelectasis*. When the lungs become infected, this is called *pneumonia*.

In order to keep your lungs clear and open as much as possible, you'll be given a device that will help to inflate all the air sacs in your lungs. This device is called a *spirometer.* You'll be given one of your own and shown how to use it, and it'll be your responsibility to do exactly that. Your lungs will thank you.

To use the spirometer, you'll put the tube in your mouth and inhale deeply, trying to lift up the gauge on the spirometer. The goal is not to hit the gauge to the top of the spirometer but to hold it up for at least 3 seconds. Repeating that process will inflate all those tiny sacs in your lungs, and more healing oxygen will be available to your body. Your doctor will expect you to do this at least ten times every hour while you're awake. Take it home and keep using it for a few days. A good time to do this is during the commercials while watching TV.

When you first start to use the spirometer, it hurts. You're stretching your lungs and forcing open the little air sacs in the lungs. But over the time you spend in the hospital, you'll be able to get that gauge to rise, and it won't be painful.

Taking advantage of physical therapy

If you're having any difficulty moving following your surgery, ask your doctor to refer you for an appointment with the occupational therapist while you're in the hospital. An occupational therapist's job is to enhance your ability to function productively and effectively in your everyday living environment. Your occupational therapist will work with you to help you improve whatever you spend your time and energy doing.

The occupational therapist will provide you with devices and teach you methods that will make moving around, picking up objects, and even dressing much easier. He can teach you how to more comfortably get out of bed and out of chairs. Your occupational therapist is accustomed to working with severely obese patients and can teach you methods that will add to your independence. Some of the devices he can offer you include the following:

- A long-handled plastic device for putting on socks
- A long-handled shoehorn to help you get your shoes on without putting undue pressure on your abdomen
- Different long-handled devices that will help you bathe, groom, keep clean, and use the toilet
- Shower chairs, tub chairs, and raised toilet seats
- Long-handled grabbers to help you if you drop something or to help you put on your clothing without having to bend or twist

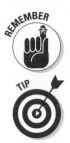

These devices are not meant to keep you from moving. They're designed to help you accomplish everyday tasks pain-free.

If you live alone, discuss with your surgeon the possibility of being discharged from the hospital to the rehabilitation department rather than going directly home. You'll be able to ease into moving around, especially if you've had a little longer hospital stay because of any complications. After such major surgery and the dizzying effects of anesthesia, you may not be as steady on your feet as you'd like. You want to be steady and safe before going home. The rehabilitation therapist will work with you on movement, balance, and flexibility. She'll show you various exercises to do to start you on the road to better mobility. And she'll have you up and walking, walking, walking.

Making the Trip Home

Be sure to arrange to have a ride home from the hospital. As much as you're looking forward to going home, the trip can be an uncomfortable experience. You'll be dealing with seat belts, the abdominal strain of getting in and out of the car, and the inevitable bumps along the way. You also may feel dizziness and nausea from the anesthesia.

If you live near the hospital, here are some tips to make going home a bit more bearable:

- ✔ **Wear very loose clothing.** Wearing clothing that puts any pressure on your abdomen will be painful. Make sure your clothes are very loose fitting, with a stretchy waistband.

- ✔ **Time your pain medication so you take a dose just before leaving the hospital.**

- ✔ **Have a pillow with you in the car so you can hold it against your abdomen for support.**

- ✔ **Take a bottle of water with you so you can sip all the way home.** This will help you avoid dehydration — and help you develop the habit of drinking enough water.

- ✔ **Do ankle exercises by flexing your feet back and forth and then rotating each foot in a circle.**

If you have a long drive home, do all the preceding but also stop every hour and stretch. Find a rest stop or restaurant and walk around. Getting out of the car and moving around will help prevent the possibility of blood clots forming in your legs. You won't be able to drive for a week to ten days, so don't expect to share any of the driving. And definitely don't even consider driving if you're still using your pain medication.

If your trip home is by airplane, you're most likely a week to ten days post-op because you've stayed the extra time in a hotel after your hospital discharge. Although an exit row would be the most comfortable, you won't be fit and strong enough to help out in an emergency (a requirement of the airlines), so you won't be able to sit there.

Sitting in first class is your best bet if it's available on your flight and if you can afford it. If first class isn't an option, ask for an aisle seat so you can easily stand up and walk around without having to climb over anyone. As embarrassing as it may be, ask for a seat-belt extender. Remind yourself that this may very well be the last time you'll have to do that.

Take advantage of the airport escort service and use a wheelchair to get around the airport. Although walking is very important, the walk in the airport with a carry-on bag may be too strenuous at this point.

Chapter 10

Knowing What You Can Eat for the First Few Months

After your surgery, you'll need to make permanent changes in the way you eat, including limiting the amount you eat at any one time. At first, some of these adjustments are difficult. But keep in mind that they're essential for successful weight loss and a healthier life.

Your diet will start off with clear liquids. Then you'll progress to full liquids; then to pureed foods; and finally to solid foods. (In this chapter, we take you through the first few stages; we cover solid foods in Chapter 11.) Each stage is designed to give you what you need nutritionally, as well as to help you lose weight safely and effectively. It also gives you a chance to heal internally while getting familiar with your new stomach, whether it's the small stomach above the band, the gastric pouch in a Roux-en-Y bypass, or the smaller stapled stomach in a sleeve gastrectomy or duodenal switch.

After your surgery, your new stomach will be swollen. Gradually moving from liquids to solid foods is a way of preventing discomfort and vomiting. You want to make sure your new stomach isn't stretched too much, because that can cause leaks. As you can probably guess, if the contents of your stomach leak into other areas of your body, this can cause serious health issues and even death.

Different foods and drinks empty your stomach at different rates. Liquids empty your new stomach the quickest, followed by soft foods, and then solid foods. The more solid and dense the food you're taking in, the longer you'll feel full. If you keep this information in mind, you can gear your eating to help you avoid hunger. Even though you won't feel hunger for a while, and you can't jump to solid foods right away, you eventually will, and you'll be able to use this information to help you feel full.

Be sure to stay in each dietary stage for the length of time your surgeon requires. When you follow the stages as prescribed by your surgeon, liquid and softer foods will empty your new stomach more easily, and you'll have less chance of vomiting. Your dietitian can assist you in understanding and adjusting to these guidelines.

This chapter covers general dietary guidelines for people who've had weight loss surgery. Eating guidelines vary from surgeon to surgeon, as well as for each type of procedure. The guidelines in this chapter should not be a substitute for your own surgeon's guidelines. When in doubt, always go with what your surgeon says.

Stage 1: Clear Liquids

Immediately after your weight loss surgery, on the day of the surgery itself, you may not be allowed to have anything to drink, and you definitely won't be allowed to have anything to eat. Your surgeon *may* allow you to have ice chips.

Stage 1, which is the clear-liquid stage, starts the day after your surgery. Clear liquids are any liquids you can see through — but before you go getting any funny ideas, you should know that this doesn't include alcoholic beverages. In addition to good old H_2O, now you can expand your palate to include

- High-protein broth (chicken or beef)
- Sugar-free gelatin
- Sugar-free ice pops
- Decaffeinated tea
- Crystal Light
- Sugar-free Kool-Aid
- Sugar-free Tang
- Juices you can see through

You may have some problems with juices, because they're high in sugar. Most surgeons discourage their patients from drinking juice. If you're sick of water, though, and you want more flavor, diluting juice with a lot of water is okay. Some people like to use apple juice, but others find it so sweet that it makes them nauseated. Orange juice and tomato juice are acidic and not considered clear liquids. Many patients like a cranberry juice mixture sweetened with Splenda so it's lower in sugar. Think one part juice to nine parts water for a little flavor.

Your main goal in this stage is to stay properly hydrated, so try to drink 2 or 3 ounces every 30 minutes. Keep sipping as much as you can tolerate. You may be surprised by how difficult it is to drink enough fluids after surgery. Generally, 64 ounces of fluids per day is a minimum. (***Note:*** When we say *fluids,* we mean low-calorie, caffeine-free liquids.)

Right after surgery, many patients are constipated. If you experience constipation, you'll need to drink fluids, fluids, and more fluids. Constipation usually is caused by dehydration. Drinking enough clear liquids is the best thing you can do to prevent this from happening. Your doctor may suggest a gentle stimulant such as milk of magnesia after making sure that you're adequately hydrated.

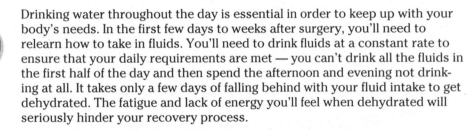

Drinking water throughout the day is essential in order to keep up with your body's needs. In the first few days to weeks after surgery, you'll need to relearn how to take in fluids. You'll need to drink fluids at a constant rate to ensure that your daily requirements are met — you can't drink all the fluids in the first half of the day and then spend the afternoon and evening not drinking at all. It takes only a few days of falling behind with your fluid intake to get dehydrated. The fatigue and lack of energy you'll feel when dehydrated will seriously hinder your recovery process.

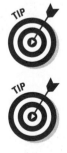

When you notice you're feeling sluggish, take in more clear liquids. Additional side effects of dehydration include dizziness, dry skin, and headaches. Be aware that caffeine can contribute to dehydration, so avoid caffeinated beverages whenever possible. Remember to take extra caution during hot weather.

The color of your urine can provide a good clue as to whether you're drinking enough liquids. Your urine should be pale yellow or clear. If it's dark yellow (and if you aren't taking a medication or vitamin that colors your urine), you need to drink more water.

Don't wait until you're thirsty to drink. By the time you begin to feel parched, your body has already started to dehydrate. Drink water or other beverages in small, frequent sips throughout the day. Always carry a water bottle with you wherever you go.

Your new stomach will fill with liquids quickly and empty slowly. That's why sipping is so important. Don't use straws — they can cause you to swallow a lot of air, which can cause gas. Also, be sure not to gulp too soon after surgery, for the same reason. Here are a couple ways to slow yourself down:

- ✔ Freeze water bottles overnight and sip them the next day while they're melting.
- ✔ Set your cup down after each swallow.
- ✔ Use children's sippy cups.

Make sure you can tolerate clear liquids before moving on to the next stage. Your surgeon will let you know whether you're ready. When in doubt, ask.

Stage 2: Full Liquids and Thin Purees

Stage 2, the full-liquid stage, may start as early as the second day after your surgery, or it may start as many as two weeks to a month after surgery. Your surgeon is the one who decides when to start you on Stage 2 — remember to follow your surgeon's guidelines over anyone else's.

Some surgeons consider the full-liquid stage as part of the puree diet; for this book, we've made Stage 2 full liquids and thin purees, and Stage 3 thicker purees.

In this stage, you can have everything you had in Stage 1, plus the following:

- ✔ Strained or pureed soups
- ✔ Broths
- ✔ Skim or 1 percent milk
- ✔ Low-fat soy milk
- ✔ Buttermilk
- ✔ Lactaid (lactose-free milk)
- ✔ Water-based protein supplement
- ✔ Protein shakes
- ✔ Sugar-free pudding or custard (You can add unflavored protein powder like Unjury for more nutrition.)
- ✔ Hot cereals (thin and soupy), Cream of Wheat, Cream of Rice, or oatmeal

✔ Light yogurt (Choose smooth yogurts, not yogurt with fruit on the bottom that needs to be mixed in. Light yogurts are those that have less than 100 calories per serving.)

✔ The yolk of a soft-boiled egg

Only 8 to 12 ounces of your total fluid intake will come from these liquid meals. The other 52 to 56 ounces should be low-calorie, noncarbonated, clear fluids, such as water or Crystal Light. You'll be consuming between 300 and 600 calories per day and remain in Stage 2 for approximately two weeks, or until your surgeon advises you to advance to the next stage.

Some patients have a difficult time drinking liquids that are too hot or too cold. Take things very slowly, paying close attention to how your body responds.

Mix powdered skim milk into regular milk to create a protein-dense base. Then mix the base with low-fat creamed soups (cream of chicken, potato, and so on).

For at least the first one to two months after surgery, have any of the following foods or beverages with caution and after talking to your surgeon, because they can cause stomach irritation and discomfort:

✔ Caffeinated beverages

✔ Carbonated beverages

✔ Citrus juices

✔ Raw fruits (except bananas) and raw vegetables

✔ Sugar and other sugar sweeteners, including the following (predominantly for bypass patients):

- Dextrin

- Dextrose

- High-fructose corn syrup

- Fructose

- Fruit juice concentrate

- Glactose

- Lactose

- Maltose

- Mannitol

- Polyol

- Sorghum

- Sucrose

- Turbinado

There is a big difference between "sugar-free" and "no sugar added." Bypass patients may be very sensitive to any sweetness following surgery. "No sugar added" may *sound* harmless, but a "no-sugar-added" food or drink may have a high *natural sugar* content, and it can make you very nauseated. Proceed with caution.

Table 10-1 provides a typical menu for a Stage 2 thin-puree diet. As always, if your surgeon advises something other than what we list here, follow the menu recommended by your surgeon.

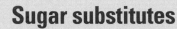

Sugar substitutes

Most sugar substitutes are low in calories and can be useful in lowering your caloric intake. Keep in mind that foods that contain sugar substitutes aren't necessarily lower in calories than similar products that contain sugars. Make sure you read labels carefully.

The following is a list of some of the more popular sugar substitutes:

- **Acesulfame-K:** Found in Sunette and Sweet One. This is a synthetic chemical and is noncaloric, because your body can't metabolize it.

- **Agave nectar:** A natural sweetener made from the leaves of the agave plant. Ounce per ounce, agave nectar is up to two times sweeter than sugar, so less agave nectar is needed to sweeten your drinks.

- **Aspartame:** Found in Equal and NutraSweet. This is a synthetic derivative of a combination of the amino acids aspartic acid and phenylalanine. It has 4 calories per gram, but only tiny amounts are needed to sweeten food, so it's considered calorie-free.

- **Saccharin:** Found in Sweet'N Low. This synthetic was discovered more the 100 years ago. Your body can't break it down, so it's considered calorie-free.

- **Stevia:** Also known as Truvia. This natural sugar substitute is made from the leaves of plants in the *Stevia* genus. Stevia is much sweeter than sugar, so less is needed. In addition, stevia does not cause the same rise in blood sugar that sugar does.

- **Sucralose:** Found in Splenda. This is the only low-calorie sweetener that is made from sugar. Sugar (sucrose) is chemically combined with chlorine. It's low calorie because your body can't burn sucralose for energy.

- **Sugar alcohols:** Also known as *sorbitol, xylitol,* and *mannitol.* These substances are made by adding hydrogen atoms to sugars. Your body absorbs them slowly and incompletely. A side effect for some people, especially if large amounts of sugar alcohols are consumed, is diarrhea. They don't raise blood sugar as rapidly as regular sugar, but some are caloric.

- **Tagatose:** Also known as Naturlose. A mirror image of sugar manufactured from lactose. The enzymes in your intestines do not digest tagatose, so it's considered calorie free.

Table 10-1   **Adjustable Gastric Band Stage 2 (Thin Puree) Diet**

	Day 1	Day 2	Day 3	Day 4	Day 5	Day 6
Breakfast	1 scoop protein powder, 1 cup nonfat milk, ¼ cup sliced frozen strawberries	6 ounces sugar-free yogurt, ¼ cup unsweetened applesauce	6 ounces Cream of Wheat, 1 cup nonfat milk	2 poached eggs	1 scoop protein powder, 1 cup nonfat milk, 1 small banana	6 ounces sugar-free yogurt
Lunch	1 slice cheese, 1 cup mashed cauliflower, 1 teaspoon margarine	2 eggs whisked and boiled in 1 cup chicken broth	1 cup tomato soup, ½ cup string beans blended	1 cup leek soup made with nonfat milk	1 cup blended fat-free Healthy Choice soup (cream of broccoli, mushroom, or chicken)	½ cup 1 percent cottage cheese, ½ cup unsweetened applesauce
Snack	½ cup sugar-free yogurt	1 scoop protein powder, 1 cup nonfat milk	1 scoop protein powder, 1 cup nonfat milk	½ cup part-skim ricotta cheese; drop of vanilla extract; 1 packet Splenda; cinnamon	½ cup diet pudding	1 scoop protein powder, 1 cup nonfat milk
Dinner	1 cup miso soup, ½ cup blended broccoli, 1 teaspoon margarine	1 cup split pea soup, ¼ cup mashed potato	½ cup 1 percent cottage cheese, ½ cup unsweetened applesauce	1 cup Lipton chicken noodle soup, 2 tablespoons tofu added	1 cup egg drop soup, ½ cup blended string beans	1 cup chicken soup, 1 slice skim mozzarella cheese melted
Daily Total	630 calories, 18g fat, 76g cholesterol, 45g protein	706 calories, 18g fat, 80g cholesterol, 47g protein	600 calories, 12g fat, 87g cholesterol, 50g protein	642 calories, 25g fat, 66g cholesterol, 44g protein	600 calories, 16g fat, 82g cholesterol, 50g protein	594 calories, 12g fat, 64g cholesterol, 56g protein

Stage 3: Purees

Stage 3 is the puree stage. As we mention in the preceding section, some surgeons combine full liquids with purees in one stage — in this book, we divide them into separate stages, but as always, follow your doctor's recommendations.

Some people find it more convenient to use stage-one baby foods instead of creating their own purees. If you prefer to make your own purees, you can mix foods like lean meats in the blender until they're notably soft and smooth in consistency. Adding nonfat milk, juice, or water to pureed food can make it easier to swallow. Pureed fruits, vegetables, and smoothies also are suitable at this stage.

At this stage, you're eating only 2 ounces (¼ cup) of food, two to three times per day. You may be able to eat a little more if you've had gastric banding surgery.

To ensure you're getting enough protein, your surgeon may recommend a protein powder supplement that can be mixed with water. In this section, we provide some protein shake recipes that you can try as well.

Protein sources in this stage include

- Scrambled eggs
- No-sugar-added or light yogurt
- Part-skim ricotta cheese
- Stage-one baby food meats
- Low-fat, small-curd cottage cheese
- Pureed chicken, fish, or tofu

You may experience discomfort when eating meat and milk products after surgery. If so, your surgeon will have you use another protein source, possibly a protein supplement.

Try to take in 1.5 grams of protein per kilogram of your weight every day (or about 0.68 grams of protein per pound of your weight). This will help maximize your weight loss and preserve muscle mass. Early on in your weight loss journey, this means drinking protein shakes to get that amount of protein in every day.

Suitable food choices in the carbohydrate category include

- ✔ Smooth oatmeal
- ✔ Cream of Wheat
- ✔ Cream of Rice
- ✔ Stage-one baby food vegetables and fruits
- ✔ Pureed vegetables and pureed fruits

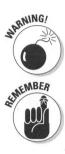

Don't use the prepackaged oatmeal (it's high in sugar). Instead, cook your own oatmeal and add a sugar substitute like Splenda to make it more palatable.

Carbohydrates should be a very minimal part of your diet throughout these stages and for the rest of your life because of your body's protein requirements. Your body needs carbohydrates mainly for energy. The best sources are whole grains such as oatmeal, whole-wheat bread, and long-grain brown rice.

You'll normally be in this stage for two weeks, unless your surgeon advises otherwise.

Do not advance to the next stage on your own. Remaining in each stage for the amount of time your surgeon requires is important. Advancing on your own, even if you feel you can tolerate more solid types of food, can be very dangerous. If something gets stuck, you're in for four to six hours of misery that no one, including your surgeon, can help you with. (You can try to burp it up or sip a little warm water with meat tenderizer dissolved in it. Chapter 11 has other tips on early eating strategies.)

Try your hand at the recipes later in this section if you're looking for some variety. Typical menus for a Stage 3 thin-puree diet are shown in Table 10-2 (for someone who's had Roux-en-Y gastric bypass or sleeve gastrectomy surgery) and Table 10-3 (for someone who's had gastric band surgery). As always, follow the menu recommended by your surgeon over what we list here.

Note: We call for Unjury in some of the recipes in this chapter. Unjury is a brand name of a protein supplement. You can use other supplements if you can't find Unjury, but you may need to make some adjustments according to taste.

Table 10-2   Roux-en-Y Gastric Bypass/Sleeve Gastrectomy Stage 3 (Puree) Diet

	Day 1	Day 2	Day 3	Day 4	Day 5	Day 6
Breakfast	½ cup nonfat milk, 1 pouch Cream of Wheat	¼ cup 1 percent cottage cheese, ¼ cup unsweetened applesauce	1 egg poached, 1 ounce cheese	½ cup oatmeal, ¼ cup sliced banana	1 egg scrambled, ¼ cup salsa	1 pouch Cream of Wheat, ½ cup nonfat milk
Protein	8 ounces protein supplement	8 ounces protein supplement	8 ounces protein supplement	8 ounces protein supplement	8 ounces protein supplement	8 ounces protein supplement
Lunch	4 ounces Dannon fruit blends, 1 ounce canned peaches	1 can light cream of chicken soup	1 can tomato soup	¼ cup beans, 2 tablespoons avocado puree, ¼ cup salsa	3 ounces part-skim ricotta cheese, vanilla extract, Equal	3 ounces puree chicken, 1 ounce mashed potato, 2 tablespoons peas or carrots
Protein	8 ounces protein supplement	8 ounces protein supplement	8 ounces protein supplement	8 ounces protein supplement	8 ounces protein supplement	8 ounces protein supplement
Dinner	½ cup refried beans, 1 ounce cheese	2 ounces cod fish, 1 cup mashed yam	2 ounces chicken salad, 1 cup green beans	3 ounces tuna salad	1 can split pea soup	2 ounces Dinty Moore Beef Stew, 1 ounce mashed potato, 2 tablespoons peas or carrots
Optional	Diet gelatin	4 ounces Dannon fruit blends	Diet gelatin	4 ounces nonfat milk	4 ounces protein supplement	4 ounces. Dannon fruit blends
Daily Total	736 calories, 19g fat, 10g saturated fat, 92g cholesterol, 1,826mg sodium, 16g fiber, 68g protein	737 calories, 21g fat, 7g saturated fat, 83g cholesterol, 2,394mg sodium, 13g fiber, 66g protein	687 calories, 31g fat, 12g saturated fat, 56g cholesterol, 3,036mg sodium, 11g fiber, 62g protein	737 calories, 27g fat, 9g saturated fat, 70g cholesterol, 1,130mg sodium, 19g fiber, 75g protein	770 calories, 37g fat, 18g saturated fat, 65g cholesterol, 2,500mg sodium, 13g fiber, 78g protein	641 calories, 24g fat, 9g saturated fat, 55g cholesterol, 1,122mg sodium, 9g fiber, 64g protein

Table 10-3   **Adjustable Gastric Band Stage 3 (Puree) Diet**

	Day 1	Day 2	Day 3	Day 4	Day 5	Day 6
Breakfast	1 scoop protein powder, 1 cup nonfat milk, 1 packet hot cereal	6 ounces sugar-free yogurt, ¼ cup unsweetened apple-sauce	½ cup 1 percent cottage cheese, ½ cup unsweetened canned peaches (mashed)	2 poached eggs	1 scoop protein powder, 1 cup nonfat milk, 1 small banana	1 scoop protein powder, 1 cup nonfat milk, 1 packet hot cereal
Lunch	½ cup tuna with low-fat mayonnaise, ½ cup split pea soup	½ cup egg salad with low-fat mayonnaise, ½ cup tomato soup	1 cup blended soup, ½ cup string beans blended	½ cup fat-free refried beans, ¼ cup tomato salsa	1 cup blended fat-free Healthy Choice soup (cream of broccoli, mushroom, or chicken)	½ cup 1 percent cottage cheese, ½ cup unsweetened canned peaches (mashed)
Snack	½ cup sugar-free yogurt	1 scoop protein powder, 1 cup nonfat milk	½ cup diet pudding	½ cup part-skim ricotta cheese; drop of vanilla extract; 1 packet Splenda, cinnamon	½ cup diet pudding	½ cup sugar-free yogurt
Dinner	½ cup crustless quiche, ½ cup blended broccoli florets, 1 teaspoon margarine	3 ounces tender fish, ¼ cup mashed cooked carrots, 1 teaspoon margarine	½ cup crustless quiche, ½ cup mashed potato, 1 teaspoon margarine	1 cup potato leek soup made with nonfat milk	3 ounces tuna with low-fat mayo, 2 ounces creamed spinach	3 ounces tender fish poached, 1 slice skim mozzarella cheese, melted
Daily Total	720 calories, 28g fat, 90g cholesterol, 60g protein	816 calories, 28g fat, 80g cholesterol, 58g protein	700 calories, 32g fat, 97g cholesterol, 60g protein	762 calories, 28g fat, 92g cholesterol, 54g protein	770 calories, 32g fat, 92g cholesterol, 68g protein	800 calories, 28g fat, 74g cholesterol, 70g protein

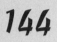

Chocolate-Covered Cherries Shake

Stage: 3 • **Prep time:** About 5 min • **Cook time:** 0 min • **Yield:** 1 serving (9 ounces)

Ingredients	*Instructions*
2 scoops Unjury chocolate	Place all ingredients into a blender and blend until smooth.
4 ounces skim milk, frozen into cubes	
2 ounces plain, low-fat yogurt	
2 ounces skim milk	
1 ounce fresh cherries, pitted	

Per serving: Calories 299 (From Fat 11); Fat 1g (Saturated 1g); Cholesterol 7mg; Sodium 238mg; Carbohydrate 24g (Dietary Fiber 0g); Protein 49g.

Tip: You can use frozen cherries if you can't find fresh.

Chocolate Peanut Butter Shake

Stage: 3 • **Prep time:** About 5 min • **Cook time:** 0 min • **Yield:** 1 serving (8 ounces)

Ingredients	*Instructions*
2 scoops Unjury chocolate	Place all ingredients into a blender and blend until smooth.
4 ounces skim milk, frozen into cubes	
4 ounces skim milk	
1 tablespoon peanut butter	
1 package sugar substitute	

Per serving: Calories 358 (From Fat 77); Fat 9g (Saturated 2g); Cholesterol 5mg; Sodium 303mg; Carbohydrate 21g (Dietary Fiber 1g); Protein 52g.

Vary It! If you'd like to try something a little different, look for other nut butters, such as almond butter or cashew butter. You can find these at most health-food stores.

Orange Creamsicle Shake

Stage: 3 • **Prep time:** About 5 min • **Cook time:** 0 min • **Yield:** 1 serving (9 ounces)

Ingredients	Instructions
4 ounces skim milk, frozen into cubes	Place all ingredients into a blender (in the order listed) and blend until smooth.
1 ounce mandarin oranges, drained	
4 ounces plain low-fat yogurt	
2 scoops Unjury vanilla	
1 packet sugar substitute	

Per serving: Calories 306 (From Fat 18); Fat 2g (Saturated 1g); Cholesterol 9mg; Sodium 250mg; Carbohydrate 23g (Dietary Fiber 0g); Protein 50g.

Tip: Other varieties of oranges will not mix well in the blender and will cause the shake to become stringy and undrinkable. If you want to substitute orange juice for the mandarin oranges, you can do so, but keep in mind that the recipe won't contain the needed fiber.

Vanilla Cappuccino Shake

Stage: 3 • **Prep time:** About 5 min • **Cook time:** 0 min • **Yield:** 1 serving (8 ounces)

Ingredients	Instructions
2 scoops Unjury vanilla	Place all ingredients into a blender and blend until smooth.
4 ounces skim milk, frozen into cubes	
4 ounces skim milk	
1 tablespoon instant coffee, decaffeinated	
½ teaspoon vanilla extract	
1 packet sugar substitute	

Per serving: Calories 280 (From Fat 4); Fat 0g (Saturated 0g); Cholesterol 5mg; Sodium 229mg; Carbohydrate 20g (Dietary Fiber 0g); Protein 48g.

Vary It! Instead of vanilla extract, you can use almond extract for a nutty flavor. To make a mocha cappuccino, use Unjury chocolate protein powder.

Strawberry and Banana Smoothie

Stage: 3 • **Prep time:** About 5 min • **Cook time:** 0 min • **Yield:** 1 serving (9 ounces)

Ingredients	Instructions
2 scoops Unjury vanilla	Place all ingredients into a blender and blend until smooth.
4 ounces skim milk, frozen into cubes	
4 ounces plain low-fat yogurt	
½ ounce strawberries, stems removed	
½ ounce banana, sliced	
1 packet sugar substitute	
½ teaspoon vanilla extract	

Per serving: Calories 317 (From Fat 19); Fat 2g (Saturated 1g); Cholesterol 9mg; Sodium 249mg; Carbohydrate 25g (Dietary Fiber 1g); Protein 50g.

Tip: If you can't find fresh strawberries, you can use frozen ones.

Vary It! For an even thicker shake, use frozen bananas and strawberry pieces. You also can try other berries, such as raspberries and blueberries.

Dealing with monotony

Don't rush yourself. Be patient as you're going through the various stages. Remember that you aren't always going to eat this way. In a year, you'll probably be able to eat almost anything, just in smaller quantities. Give your new system time to adjust.

If you're eating the same foods over and over again, you can become very bored with what you're eating. But as you can see from the menus and recipes in this chapter, with some imagination and creativity, you can have very interesting and satisfying meals regardless of what stage you're in.

Dreamy Seafood Salad

Stage: 3 • **Prep time:** About 5 min • **Cook time:** 0 min • **Yield:** 4 servings (4 ounces each)

Ingredients	Instructions
8 ounces crab meat, cooked	*1* Place all ingredients, except lime wedge, into a food processor.
4 ounces cooked shrimp, peeled and deveined	
4 ounces scallops, cooked	*2* Blend for 20 seconds and, using a plastic rubber spatula, scrape the sides of the bowl.
¼ cup cocktail sauce	
2 tablespoons light sour cream	*3* Puree for an additional 35 seconds. Garnish with a lime wedge and serve.
1 teaspoon onion powder	
2 teaspoons lime juice	
2 cloves fresh garlic	
Lime wedge (for garnish)	

Per serving: Calories 166 (From Fat 19); Fat 2g (Saturated 1g); Cholesterol 137mg; Sodium 584mg; Carbohydrate 6g (Dietary Fiber 0g); Protein 28g.

Tip: Store this spread in an airtight container. It will keep its freshness for two days.

Note: If you have to clean and devein your own shrimp, check out Figure 10-1 for guidelines.

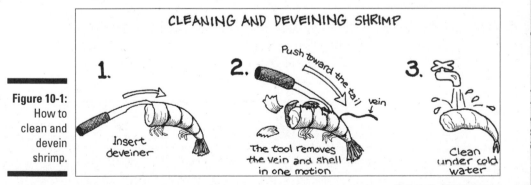

Figure 10-1: How to clean and devein shrimp.

CLEANING AND DEVEINING SHRIMP

1. Insert deveiner

2. Push toward the tail — vein — The tool removes the vein and shell in one motion

3. Clean under cold water

Illustration by Elizabeth Kurtzman

Egg Salad

Stage: 3 • **Prep time:** About 10 min • **Cook time:** 0 min • **Yield:** 4 servings (3 ounces each)

Ingredients	Instructions
6 large eggs, hard-boiled and peeled	**1** Slice the eggs in half and remove the yolks.
½ teaspoon celery seed, chopped	**2** Place the whites in the food processor until very finely diced. Remove.
1 teaspoon fresh lemon juice	**3** Place the egg yolks, celery seed, and lemon juice into a food processor.
¼ cup light sour cream	**4** Puree for 20 seconds.
¼ cup light mayonnaise	**5** Using a rubber spatula, scrape down the sides of the bowl.
Salt and pepper, to taste	**6** Add the sour cream, mayonnaise, salt, and pepper, and puree for another 30 seconds.
	7 Fold the finely diced egg whites into the mixture. Serve.

Per serving: Calories 188 (From Fat 128); Fat 14g (Saturated 4g); Cholesterol 328mg; Sodium 391mg; Carbohydrate 4g (Dietary Fiber 0g); Protein 10g.

Tip: Store this spread in an airtight container. It will keep its freshness for two days.

How much can you eat?

You'll be able to eat more with time. In case you're curious, here are the amounts you can eat after gastric bypass and sleeve gastrectomy:

- **1 month:** 1 to 1½ ounces (2 to 3 tablespoons)
- **3 months:** 3 ounces (¼ cup)
- **6 months:** 4 to 5 ounces (½ cup)
- **18 to 24 months:** 8 to 10 ounces (1 to 1¼ cup)

With gastric banding and biliopancreatic diversion with duodenal switch, you can eat about ½ cup at two weeks and 1 cup at one month. With band adjustments, this amount will decrease.

Garlic Chicken Salad

Stage: 3 • Prep time: About 5 min • Cook time: 0 min • Yield: 4 servings (4 ounces each)

Ingredients	*Instructions*
1 pound cooked chicken, with fat and skin removed	*1* Place all ingredients except the chicken stock into a food processor.
1 tablespoon olive oil	*2* Puree for 30 seconds.
2 tablespoons apple cider vinegar	
1 teaspoon onion powder	*3* Using a rubber spatula, scrape down the sides of the bowl.
1 teaspoon garlic powder	
Salt and pepper, to taste	*4* Add half the chicken stock and puree for 15 seconds.
2 teaspoons chopped fresh basil	*5* Add the remaining chicken stock and blend for another 15 seconds.
¼ cup chicken stock	

Per serving: Calories 253 (From Fat 108); Fat 12g (Saturated 3g); Cholesterol 101mg; Sodium 306mg; Carbohydrate 1g (Dietary Fiber 0g); Protein 33g.

Tip: Store this spread in an airtight container. It will keep its freshness for two days.

Tip: If you like chicken salad thicker, add less stock; if you prefer it thinner, add more chicken stock.

White Albacore Tuna Spread

Stage: 3 • **Prep time:** About 12 min • **Cook time:** 0 min • **Yield:** 2 servings (4 ounces each)

Ingredients	*Instructions*
7 ounces white albacore tuna in a pouch	**1** Place the tuna, dill, hot sauce, garlic, and lemon juice in a 3-cup food processor.
2 tablespoons fresh dill weed, chopped	**2** Puree for 20 seconds. Using a rubber spatula, scrape down the sides of the bowl.
1 teaspoon hot sauce	
1 teaspoon garlic, minced	**3** Add the sour cream, mayonnaise, salt, and pepper, and puree for another 30 seconds. Garnish with fresh dill and lemon wedge, and serve.
1 tablespoon fresh lemon juice	
¼ cup light sour cream	
¼ cup light mayonnaise	
Salt and pepper, to taste	
Fresh dill (for garnish)	
Lemon wedge (for garnish)	

Per serving: Calories 272 (From Fat 139); Fat 16g (Saturated 4g); Cholesterol 62mg; Sodium 1,033mg; Carbohydrate 6g (Dietary Fiber 0g); Protein 25g.

Tip: Store this spread in an airtight container. It will keep its freshness for two days.

Nice and warm

In the first few months following my surgery, it would take me so long to eat that my food would get cold. I would try to reheat my food in the microwave, but it would turn dry and rubbery. I discovered that if I put my food on a small saucer from a teacup and placed it on an electric mug warmer, it would keep my food hot and moist the whole time while I ate. I have a warmer for my home and my office, and I never have to eat cold or rubbery food again!

Stacy Leary
Rochester, New Hampshire

Stage 4: Soft Foods

Stage 4 is the soft-food stage. (Some programs consider this a separate stage, and others consider it part of the puree stage.) At this point, you start to get a little more variety. Protein sources include

- Finely ground tuna
- Chicken salad or egg salad with low-fat mayonnaise (no celery or onion)
- Shrimp
- Scallops
- White fish (no need to puree or chop up)

At this stage, you can have vegetables that are well cooked, but not pureed. You also can add to your diet, on a limited basis, "light" canned fruits, packed in their own juice, such as peaches, pears, or fruit cocktail. *Remember:* Fruits and vegetables are complex carbohydrates, which is the type you should be having, but still only in limited amounts.

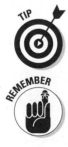

When adding new foods, try a spoonful at a time so you can figure out whether it bothers you. Don't try more than one new food every couple days. Be prepared for the fact that you'll tolerate a food very well one day and not the next.

Sometimes, you may feel as though you're taking one step forward and two steps back. Don't get discouraged. It just takes time.

You're in this stage for approximately two weeks.

Typical menus for a Stage 4 soft food diet are shown in Table 10-4. As always, follow the menu recommended by your surgeon over what we list here.

Table 10-4	Stage 4 (Soft Foods) Diet					
	Day 1	**Day 2**	**Day 3**	**Day 4**	**Day 5**	**Day 6**
Breakfast	1 scrambled egg, 1 ounce shredded cheese, 1 slice whole-grain toast	½ cup old-fashioned oats, 3 tablespoons blueberries, 8 ounces nonfat milk	½ cup 1 percent cottage cheese, ¼ cup canned pears in water	½ slice whole-grain toast; 1 tablespoon peanut butter; 1 small banana, sliced	½ cup part-skim ricotta cheese, 3 tablespoons blueberries, 1 packet Splenda, ¼ teaspoon vanilla extract, cinnamon	½ cup Shredded Wheat, 8 ounces nonfat milk with 1 scoop protein powder, ¼ cup sliced strawberries
Protein	8 ounces protein supplement	8 ounces protein supplement	8 ounces protein supplement	8 ounces protein supplement	8 ounces protein supplement	8 ounces protein supplement
Lunch	3 ounces tuna salad with light mayonnaise, 1 cup baby spinach	3 thin slices Healthy Choice ham, 1 slice tomato, 1 slice whole-grain toast	3 thin slices turkey, 1 slice tomato, 1 slice whole-grain toast, Dijonnaise	½ cup egg salad with 1 teaspoon light mayonnaise, 1 slice lettuce, 1 slice tomato, 3 melba toast crackers	½ cup blended chicken salad on chopped green lettuce with tomato	½ Subway 6-inch tuna on toast or 4 crackers
Dinner	1 can chicken noodle soup, ½ small sweet potato, 1 teaspoon butter	3 ounces cooked salmon, 1 teaspoon butter, ½ cup peas and carrots, ½ cup boiled potato with skin	½ cup fat-free refried beans, 1 ounce Mexican cheese, 5 tortilla chips	3 ounces pork tenderloin, ½ cup unsweetened applesauce, ½ cup green beans	2 ounces baby shrimp salad with light mayonnaise, ¼ cup chopped broccoli, 1 ounce melted cheese	3 ounces dark-meat chicken, without skin; 2 ounces creamed spinach
Daily Total	930 calories, 27g fat, 10g saturated fat, 120g cholesterol, 4,000mg sodium, 11g fiber, 65g protein	903 calories, 22g fat, 15g saturated fat, 102g cholesterol, 1,847mg sodium, 11g fiber, 81g protein	911 calories, 42g fat, 17g saturated fat, 89g cholesterol, 3,220mg sodium, 16g fiber, 67g protein	917 calories, 35g fat, 9g saturated fat, 97g cholesterol, 949mg sodium, 15g fiber, 77g protein	723 calories, 20g fat, 8g saturated fat, 74g cholesterol, 1,662mg sodium, 9g fiber, 81g protein	827 calories, 24g fat, 10g saturated fat, 92g cholesterol, 1,877mg sodium, 10g fiber, 77g protein

Turkey Tacos

Stage: 4 • Prep time: About 10 min • Cook time: 10 min • Yield: 4 servings (4 ounces each)

Ingredients	Instructions
1 pound ground turkey	**1** In a large sauté pan sprayed with nonstick spray over medium-high heat, place the ground turkey, onion, and garlic.
¼ cup onion, peeled and chopped	
2 cloves garlic, minced	**2** Sauté for 5 minutes.
1 teaspoon cumin	
1 teaspoon chili powder	**3** Drain any fat from the pan and return to the heat.
¼ cup tomato sauce	**4** Add the cumin, chili powder, tomato sauce, salt, and pepper, and bring to a simmer. Let simmer for 5 minutes.
Salt and pepper, to taste	
Low-fat cheddar cheese (for garnish)	**5** Place the taco mixture into a food processor and blend for 20 seconds.
Light sour cream (for garnish)	**6** Using a rubber spatula, scrape down the sides of the bowl.
	7 Puree for another 30 seconds. Garnish with low-fat cheddar cheese and light sour cream, and serve.

Per serving (not including garnish): Calories 152 (From Fat 77); Fat 9g (Saturated 3g); Cholesterol 73mg; Sodium 355mg; Carbohydrate 3g (Dietary Fiber 1g); Protein 16g.

Tip: Store this spread in an airtight container. It will keep its freshness for two days.

Vary It! You can substitute ground beef or ground pork if you'd like.

Chapter 11

Starting on Solid Food

In This Chapter

▶ Transitioning into solid foods

▶ Maintaining a healthy diet and eating plan

▶ Making some new recipes

The final stage of eating after surgery is returning to solid foods. This usually starts about the fourth to sixth week after surgery. Thankfully, most weight loss surgery patients find that their hunger is greatly diminished following surgery, so waiting four to six weeks to start back on regular food probably won't be as difficult as it sounds before your surgery.

You may have no problems eating certain foods but a hard time with many others. You'll probably become familiar with bothersome eating problems like nausea, spit-ups, foam, hiccupping, gurgling, dumping, and cramping.

In this chapter, we help you make a smooth transition to solid foods, in addition to filling you in on the necessary behavior modifications you'll need to make.

Each surgeon has his own guidelines about what to eat and what foods to avoid. Following the directions of your doctor is what's important.

The Final Stage: Solid Food

Solid food is the final stage of eating after weight loss surgery. (We cover the stages *before* solid food in Chapter 10.) In this final stage, you'll begin the important process of learning new eating habits (see "Making the Transition a Smooth One," later in this chapter). For example, you'll need to chew thoroughly and eat very slowly, spending 15 to 20 minutes with each meal, and drink your fluids between, not with, your meals.

Your dietitian may suggest that you balance your menu with about 30 percent to 35 percent of your total daily calories from protein sources, 45 percent to 50 percent from complex carbohydrates, and 20 percent to 25 percent from heart-healthy fats. Or, your dietitian may suggest that your diet be higher in protein and lower in carbohydrates. ***Remember:*** Follow the advice of your surgeon and the dietitian she recommends. No matter what the breakdown of proteins, carbs, and fats, you'll typically consume 400 to 800 calories per day.

Your surgeon and dietitian may provide some helpful menus to get you started, the bariatric food guide pyramid (shown in Figure 11-1) will help you design your own daily menus. The base of the bariatric food pyramid is protein; the sources of protein are meat, fish, eggs, dairy, and legumes. Half of your daily diet should come from these protein sources.

All the recipes in this chapter work well when you've been given the green light to go on solid foods. You aren't expected to finish an entire serving — just eat until you aren't hungry.

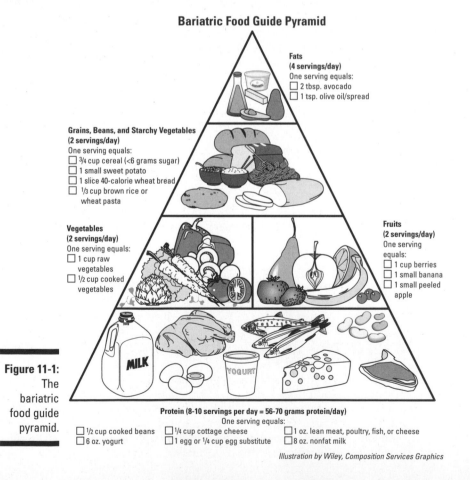

Figure 11-1:
The bariatric food guide pyramid.

Illustration by Wiley, Composition Services Graphics

Grilled Herb-Marinated Tuna with Lime

Prep time: 35 min • **Cook time:** 5 to 7 min • **Yield:** 4 servings (4 ounces each)

Ingredients	*Instructions*
2 teaspoons fresh basil, chopped	*1* Mix the herbs, lime juice, lime peel, cracked black pepper, oil, and tuna steaks together in a small bowl.
2 tablespoons fresh chives, chopped	*2* Cover and refrigerate the steaks in their herb marinade for at least 30 minutes and as long as 3 hours.
2 teaspoons fresh oregano, chopped	
2 teaspoons fresh thyme	*3* Preheat the grill.
2 tablespoons fresh squeezed lime juice	*4* Just before cooking, oil the grill by spraying it with nonstick cooking spray to keep the fish from sticking. Season the steaks with salt, and then lay the tuna steaks on the grill.
2 teaspoons lime peel	
¼ teaspoon cracked black pepper	
2 teaspoons extra-virgin olive oil	*5* Cook for 5 to 7 minutes on each side for well-done tuna or 3 minutes per side to leave a little pink in the center.
1 pound tuna steaks (about 2 small)	
½ teaspoon salt	

Per serving: Calories 143 (From Fat 30); Fat 3g (Saturated 1g); Cholesterol 49mg; Sodium 331mg; Carbohydrate 1g (Dietary Fiber 0g); Protein 26g.

Tip: We recommend fresh tuna, but you can use frozen if you prefer.

Vary It! You can broil this dish if you prefer.

Herbed Beef Patties

Prep time: About 10 min • **Cook time:** 12 min • **Yield:** 4 servings (3 ounces each)

Ingredients	*Instructions*
1 pound fresh lean ground beef 1 large egg	*1* In a large mixing bowl, combine the beef, egg, cheese, basil, oregano, thyme, garlic powder, and onion powder.
2 teaspoons Romano cheese	*2* Using your hands, form into 4 round patties.
¼ teaspoon basil	
¼ teaspoon oregano	*3* Sauté the beef patties over medium-high heat for 4 to 6 minutes, turning the patties over every 2 minutes.
¼ teaspoon thyme	
¼ teaspoon garlic powder	*4* Remove the beef patties from the sauté pan, and drain any excess fat from the pan.
¼ teaspoon onion powder	
Fresh chopped basil (for garnish)	*5* Prepare the Garlic Beef Cream Sauce, and when the sauce has started to simmer, add the cooked beef patties to the sauce and let simmer on low for 2 minutes.
	6 Garnish with fresh chopped basil and serve.

Garlic Beef Cream Sauce

2 teaspoons beef bouillon granules ¼ cup skim milk ½ cup light sour cream 1 teaspoon garlic powder Salt and pepper, to taste	In a sauté pan over medium heat, combine the beef bouillon granules and skim milk until dissolved. Add the light sour cream, garlic powder, salt, and pepper, stirring constantly until the mixture begins to lightly simmer.

Per serving: *Calories 255 (From Fat 121); Fat 13g (Saturated 6g); Cholesterol 137mg; Sodium 725mg; Carbohydrate 5g (Dietary Fiber 0g); Protein 26g.*

Tip: Stirring the sauce constantly and not letting it come to a boil are very important. If you don't, the sauce will burn and may separate.

Just-Right Chili

Prep time: About 5 min • **Cook time:** 20 min • **Yield:** 10 servings (4 ounces each)

Ingredients	Instructions
½ **pound ground beef**	*1* Place the ground beef and ground pork into a medium pot and sauté for 5 minutes.
½ **pound ground pork**	
2 teaspoons garlic, chopped	*2* Drain the fat.
½ **bunch scallions (about 2 scallions), chopped**	*3* Add the remaining ingredients and bring to a simmer; simmer for 20 minutes.
14 ounces canned tomato sauce	
14 ounces canned diced tomatoes, drained	
2 teaspoons chili powder	
1 teaspoon cumin	
½ **teaspoon black pepper**	
15-ounce can pinto beans	

Per serving: Calories 145 (From Fat 49); Fat 5g (Saturated 2g); Cholesterol 30mg; Sodium 446mg; Carbohydrate 12g (Dietary Fiber 4g); Protein 12g.

Tip: You can store this chili for up to three months in the freezer.

Vary It! You can substitute ground turkey if you prefer. You also can add Velveeta cheese to the heated chili — it makes a great dip for fresh veggies!

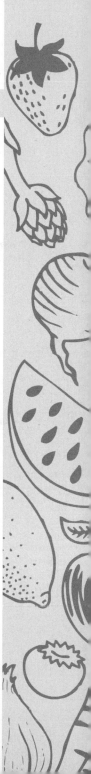

Sage Turkey Dijon Meatballs

Prep time: About 10 min • **Cook time:** 20 min • **Yield:** 5 servings (3 ounces each)

Ingredients	Instructions
1 pound ground turkey	**1** In a large mixing bowl, combine the ground turkey, sage, Italian seasoning, garlic, cheese, egg, salt, and pepper. Mix well.
2 teaspoons sage	
2 teaspoons Italian seasoning	
2 cloves garlic, minced	**2** Divide the meat mixture into 15 even pieces, and roll into 15 round balls.
¼ cup shredded Parmesan cheese	
1 large egg	**3** Spray a large sauté pan with cooking spray and heat over medium-high heat.
Salt and pepper, to taste	
¼ cup white wine	**4** When the pan is hot, add the meatballs, and sauté for 10 minutes, turning frequently to brown all sides of the meatballs.
2 tablespoons Dijon mustard	
¼ cup 2 percent milk	**5** Drain any grease from the pan, return the pan to the heat, add the white wine, and reduce by half.
½ cup light sour cream	
Chopped sage (for garnish)	**6** Add the mustard, milk, and light sour cream, and bring to a light simmer. Let simmer for 5 minutes or until meatballs have reached 165°F (74°C) in the center.
Fresh ground pepper (for garnish)	
	7 Garnish with chopped sage and fresh ground pepper, and serve.

Per serving: Calories 193 (From Fat 105); Fat 12g (Saturated 5g); Cholesterol 113mg; Sodium 500mg; Carbohydrate 5g (Dietary Fiber 1g); Protein 17g.

Tip: Be sure to stir your meatballs and sauce every 3 to 5 minutes to ensure even cooking.

Vary It! You also can use this meat mixture to make smaller meatballs for the perfect hot appetizer.

Seafood Calypso Salad

Prep time: About 10 min • **Cook time:** 0 min • **Yield:** 6 servings (4 ounces each)

Ingredients	*Instructions*
½ **pound shrimp, cooked**	**1** In a large mixing bowl, add the cooked seafood and all the ingredients.
½ **pound sea scallops, cooked**	
½ **pound crab meat, cooked**	**2** Toss well.
1 teaspoon celery seed	
1 teaspoon onion powder	**3** Place in the refrigerator and let chill for 2 hours.
2 cloves garlic, finely chopped	
1 tablespoon lime juice	**4** Garnish with lime wedges and chopped dill, and serve.
Salt and pepper, to taste	
1 tablespoon lemon juice	
½ **bunch dill, chopped (about 2 tablespoons)**	
1 teaspoon hot sauce	
¼ **cup light mayonnaise**	
¼ **cup cocktail sauce**	
Lime wedges (for garnish)	
Chopped dill (for garnish)	

Per serving: Calories 185 (From Fat 43); Fat 5g (Saturated 1g); Cholesterol 142mg; Sodium 678mg; Carbohydrate 5g (Dietary Fiber 0g); Protein 27g.

Tip: Don't use imitation crab meat; it's processed and contains less protein then real crab. Give the crab a quick rinse before cooking to be sure it's free of shells.

Vary It! You can add fresh cooked fish to this seafood dish.

Shrimp and Brie Scrambled Eggs

Prep time: About 5 min • **Cook time:** 5 min • **Yield:** 1 serving (5 ounces)

Ingredients	Instructions
2 large eggs	**1** In a small mixing bowl, mix the eggs and milk together.
1 teaspoon skim milk	
½ ounce Brie cheese	**2** Cut the Brie into small pieces and add to the egg mixture, along with the salt, pepper, and chives.
Salt and pepper, to taste	
1 teaspoon chives, minced	**3** Melt the butter in an 8-inch nonstick frying pan over medium heat.
½ teaspoon butter	
¼ cup cooked baby shrimp	**4** Place the egg mixture in the pan with the shrimp. Stir until well cooked and fluffy.

Per serving: Calories 252 (From Fat 146); Fat 16g (Saturated 7g); Cholesterol 514mg; Sodium 879mg; Carbohydrate 2g (Dietary Fiber 0g); Protein 23g.

Vary It! You can add any fish or seafood to this main-course dish. If you prefer, you can use only egg whites instead of whole eggs; just use the whites of three eggs instead.

Spicy Blue Cheese Stuffed Eggs

Prep time: About 15 min • **Cook time:** 8 min • **Yield:** 24 halves (6 servings)

Ingredients	Instructions
12 large eggs	**1** Boil eggs for 10 minutes.
½ cup crumbled blue cheese	**2** Shell then cut the eggs in half to make 24 egg halves.
3 tablespoons light mayonnaise	
3 tablespoons light sour cream	**3** Remove the yolks from the egg whites. Place the yolks in a medium mixing bowl, and add the remaining ingredients to the yolks.
1 teaspoon fresh lemon juice	
½ teaspoon Tabasco sauce	**4** Using a wire whisk, blend the ingredients well.
½ teaspoon salt	
¼ teaspoon pepper	**5** Spoon the yellow mixture back into the hollowed egg whites.
½ teaspoon celery salt	
1 tablespoon parsley, minced	

Per serving: Calories 231 (From Fat 153); Fat 17g (Saturated 6g); Cholesterol 437mg; Sodium 678mg; Carbohydrate 3g (Dietary Fiber 0g); Protein 15g.

Tip: After boiling the eggs, drop them in a pan of cold water for a few minutes. Shake them in the water to crack the shells, and then let them rest in the water for a minute or two. This usually ensures perfect peeling.

Chicken Curry Salad

Prep time: About 5 min • **Cook time:** 0 min • **Yield:** 4 servings (4 ounces each)

Ingredients	*Instructions*
1 pound cooked chicken, shredded	Place all ingredients into a large mixing bowl and mix well. Serve.
¼ cup light sour cream	
¼ cup light mayonnaise	
¼ cup golden raisins	
1 teaspoon curry powder	
½ teaspoon garlic powder	
Salt and pepper, to taste	

Per serving: Calories 321 (From Fat 133); Fat 15g (Saturated 4g); Cholesterol 111mg; Sodium 398mg; Carbohydrate 11g (Dietary Fiber 1g); Protein 34g.

Tip: For best results, purchase a rotisserie chicken from your grocery store — it tastes better than canned cooked chicken. If you're not going to eat the salad immediately, refrigerate for up to two days.

Tomato Garlic Salad

Prep time: About 10 min • **Cook time:** 0 min • **Yield:** 6 servings (3 ounces each)

Ingredients	Instructions
3 cups plum tomatoes, cut up	*1* In a large bowl, combine the tomatoes, garlic, bell pepper, cucumber, onion, and jalapeño.
2 cloves fresh garlic, minced	
½ cup green bell pepper, cut into thin strips	*2* Add the olive oil, balsamic vinegar, and Italian seasonings.
½ cup cucumber, peeled and chopped	
¼ cup red onion, finely chopped	*3* Mix well and refrigerate.
½ teaspoon fresh jalapeño pepper, minced	
¼ cup olive oil	
¼ cup balsamic vinegar	
2 teaspoons Italian seasoning	

Per serving: Calories 108 (From Fat 84); Fat 9g (Saturated 1g); Cholesterol 0mg; Sodium 9mg; Carbohydrate 6g (Dietary Fiber 1g); Protein 1g.

Tip: The longer this salad sits, the better it is.

Vary It! You can use any tomatoes in this recipe — just make sure they're as ripe as possible. Add yellow and green tomatoes to add color to this tasty dish.

Strawberry Mango Chutney

Prep time: About 10 min • **Cook time:** 0 min • **Yield:** 6 servings (3 ounces each)

Ingredients	Instructions
1 pint strawberries, stems removed and washed	**1** Place all ingredients into a food processor and blend until desired consistency.
1 large mango, peeled, seeded, and chopped	
¼ cup lime juice	**2** Chill and serve.
½ cup onion, peeled and chopped	
¼ bunch cilantro, chopped (about 2 tablespoons)	
1 clove garlic	
½ jalapeño, seeded	
Salt and pepper, to taste	

Per serving: Calories 46 (From Fat 3); Fat 0g (Saturated 0g); Cholesterol 0mg; Sodium 99mg; Carbohydrate 12g (Dietary Fiber 2g); Protein 1g.

Tip: You can store this dish in the freezer for up to three months.

Vary It! To make this chutney hotter, add more jalapeños; to make it milder, add fewer jalapeños.

Making the Transition a Smooth One

When your surgeon tells you you're finally able to start eating solid foods, you may feel like rejoicing! But instead of diving in to the water head-first, you'll want to do the equivalent of dipping your big toe in the water and seeing how it feels. In this section, we give you some insider tips on how to make your transition to solid foods a smooth one.

Keep in mind the following tips when making the transition from soft foods to solid foods:

- ✔ Don't eat raw fruits or vegetables for the first three months after your surgery.

- ✔ You may find dairy products difficult to digest. If so, you may need to switch to lactose-free dairy products for a short period of time. Don't worry — eventually you may be able to tolerate dairy again.

- ✔ Avoid anything high in sugar or fat. These foods will produce the dreaded dumping syndrome in gastric bypass patients (see Chapter 18).

- ✔ If a food doesn't agree with you at first, try it again in a few weeks.

- ✔ Make sure you're getting enough nutrition to regulate your metabolism. You may need to eat a snack to get in enough protein.

- ✔ Limit snacking between meals or scheduled snacks.

- ✔ Avoid fried foods, and limit fat.

You may have some trouble when trying to advance to solid foods. Your doctor may have you go back to liquids or purees and try solid foods again later.

If you have problems with solid food, try going back to liquids for a week and then try solid food again. But let your surgeon know about any persistent food problems. This may be a sign of a stricture or an ulcer.

Eating Guidelines to Follow from Now On

Even after you've made the transition to solid foods, you'll want to follow these dietary guidelines for the rest of your life:

- ✔ **Start each meal with a protein source.** Try to stay with dense or solid protein sources — these will keep you full longer.

- ✔ **Eat three meals each day.**

✔ **Chew your foods thoroughly.** Swallowing food in chunks may block openings and prevent food from passing. Not chewing properly also can cause nausea and vomiting. These side effects can be reduced if you:

- Chew each bite of food 20 to 30 times to the consistency of applesauce. Try practicing this before surgery. It takes longer to eat, and you'll become full with less food.

- Use small children's utensils. This strategy helps you control portion size and places less stress on your stomach after you've swallowed your food. Large bites of food will lay heavy in your new pouch and can feel uncomfortable for several hours.

- Eat slowly. Put your utensil down between bites and wait one minute between bites.

✔ **Don't overeat.** Try to tell the difference between feeling full and feeling no hunger at all. You don't want to be full after having weight loss surgery. Being full can cause nausea, a full sensation in your rib cage, and a dull pain in the middle of your chest. Stop eating just before you feel full. Also, use a saucer or a dessert plate so you don't load up your plate with food.

You want to be sure to avoid frequent vomiting, because it can lead to complications including:

- Dehydration

- Swelling of the stomach lining, which can cause an obstruction

- Possible disruption or breakdown of the staple line in the stomach or intestine

- Possible development of a hernia at the abdominal wound site

- Possible slippage or gastric prolapse in band patients

If you vomit, stop eating and drinking until the nausea passes. Repetitive vomiting to the point where liquids can't go down is potentially dangerous. If this occurs, contact your surgeon immediately. Frequent regurgitation also can lead to serious nutrient deficiencies and eating abnormalities.

It is very common to feel nausea after surgery. Slowly sipping a cup of chamomile, ginger, or peppermint tea will help sooth your stomach.

✔ **Drink between each meal, not with your meals.** Continue to drink at least 64 ounces of noncaloric fluid per day between meals.

Stop drinking fluids 30 to 45 minutes before a meal and wait at least 1 to 1½ hours after your meal before drinking again. Your new pouch is too small to allow both liquid and solid foods. Drinking too soon after a meal can overfill your pouch and cause you to feel nauseated. If the foods are too dry, add a little broth to try to moisten them.

✓ **When you're eating, ask yourself, "Will this food support good health for me?"**

✓ **Try not to talk and eat until you get accustomed to a new way of eating.**

✓ **Keep healthy foods available and get tempting unhealthy foods out of the house.**

✓ **Don't eat in front of the TV, in the car, or while you're reading.**

✓ **Take out exactly the amount of food you need to eat, and put the box or package away so you won't be tempted to eat more.**

✓ **If you're going to a party, offer to bring a healthy food item so you can be sure you'll be able to find something to eat.**

✓ **Sit up straight while you're eating.** Don't eat standing up. And if you're at a party, don't eat while standing at the food table. Take just the amount you want to eat, and go find a place to sit down with your food.

✓ **Don't go to the grocery store hungry.** Make a shopping list ahead of time and stick to the things you've written on the list — avoid impulse purchases.

✓ **Stop eating at least two or three hours before you go to bed.**

✓ **Every day, have two periods of three hours' duration during which you consume no calories.**

✓ **Pay attention to the taste of your food.** Savor each bite by becoming aware of flavor, texture, and consistency.

Your tastes may change after surgery. Foods that once were enjoyable may now taste different or no longer have the same appeal. Other foods that you disliked before surgery may become your favorites.

You also may find that food has an odd coppery taste following surgery. This coppery taste will pass in time.

✓ **Keep a journal to help yourself stay on track with your diet and liquid consumption.** Record when and where you've had a craving and what foods you craved. This exercise may teach you that specific people, places, emotions, or situations trigger your cravings — and then you can avoid those situations or be prepared going into them.

Common problem foods for gastric banding patients

Having a band in place is a constant reminder to chew your food well and pay attention while you eat. If you don't chew your food properly or if you eat foods that tend to stick together in a lump, you can experience problems. Here are some foods that can cause gastric banding patients problems depending on how much of a "fill" they have:

✔ Meat such as steak, roast beef, and pork. (Red meat is high in muscle fiber, which is tough to separate even with a tremendous amount of chewing.) Some patients can eat steak that is cooked medium rare. But the old mantra holds true: Chew, chew, chew!

✔ Dry meat.

✔ Shrimp.

✔ Untoasted bread or doughy bread.

✔ Pasta.

✔ Rice.

✔ Peanut butter.

✔ The membrane of citrus fruits.

✔ The seeds and skins of fruits and vegetables.

✔ Dried fruit.

✔ Fibrous vegetables such as corn and celery.

✔ Nuts.

✔ Coconut.

✔ Popcorn.

Chapter 12

Home Sweet Home: Returning after Surgery

Congratulations! You've had your surgery and made it to the important milestone of being released from the hospital. Getting to go home — where you're surrounded by the people and things that are familiar to you — is a joy for most patients. But as wonderful as it is to get out of the hospital, when you return home, you face new challenges, and that's what this chapter is all about.

Here, we fill you in on what to expect in those first few weeks after you get home. We also suggest ways you can get help with your kids and your housework, and we address some special considerations you may have if you live by yourself. We give you some helpful information on medications — your needs won't necessarily be the same after surgery as they were before, so expect some changes. Finally, we fill you in on post-surgery depression — a not-uncommon occurrence for weight loss surgery patients, but something you can definitely manage if you know what to expect.

Knowing What to Expect in the First Few Weeks

Being able to get out of the hospital and back to the comforts of your own home is such a reward. But when you go home, you may find yourself full of questions and a little uneasy without a team of doctors and nurses just a few steps away. In the following sections, we tell you what to expect in the first few weeks after your surgery, and we let you know what symptoms should lead you to call your doctor.

Normal feelings after surgery

Here are some typical ways that weight loss surgery patients have felt in the first weeks after surgery:

- **What have I done?** Regret is very common after surgery especially if you're struggling with nausea.

- **When am I going to wake up thin?** The months of having to lose weight yet again stretch before you. You may have incredible impatience to be thin right now.

- **What if this doesn't work for me?** There is a real concern that you won't lose any weight and that you'll fail at surgery just as you've failed at dieting.

- **I'll never be able to eat normal food again.** You will be able to eat normal food, just not as much as you used to.

- **No one knows what I'm going through.** Although your family and friends may not have been in your shoes, they are there to support you. You also can call on your surgeon or her office staff for more support.

If you experience any of these feelings, just know that you're normal — and they will go away in time.

After your surgery, you'll be eager to start losing weight, but it's important to keep in mind that each person loses weight at a different pace. Here are some factors that will influence the rate of your weight loss:

- **The amount of weight you have to lose:** If you have more weight to lose, you may lose weight at a faster rate than if you have less to lose.

- **Whether you dieted prior to surgery:** If you dieted before surgery, you may lose weight a little more slowly after your surgery. This is, in part, because you've already lost the initial water weight, so the weight you're losing following surgery is a truer weight loss.

✔ **The rate of your metabolism:** Some people have slower metabolisms than others. Men have a higher metabolic rate than women do, because men tend to have more muscle than women do. And muscle burns calories at a faster rate than fat does.

✔ **How much you're exercising:** Your physical condition will dictate how much you're able to move after surgery. The more you can get moving, the faster the weight will come off.

Each person is different. As long as you're concentrating on your own journey, you'll be okay.

When to call your surgeon

When you get home from the hospital, you'll feel weak and tired. When you drink, you may feel nausea. These feelings are completely normal. But there are other feelings that are signs that something may be wrong. If you experience any of the following symptoms, call your surgeon immediately:

✔ Excessive bleeding, swelling, or drainage from your incision

✔ Redness of your incision

✔ Unusual pain or swelling in the lower extremities

✔ Shoulder pain

✔ Body temperature above 100°F (37.7°C)

✔ Shaking or chills

✔ Increased fatigue or shortness of breath

✔ Worsening abdominal pain

✔ Inability to drink or eat

✔ Persistent nausea

✔ Excessive vomiting or frothy saliva

✔ Lightheadedness and/or fainting

✔ Black stools

✔ Blood in stools

✔ Really dark urine or no urine at all for half a day

✔ Diarrhea that is pure water

✔ A sudden increase in your drain output or a profound change in color of the fluid

✔ Any other related problems or concerns (your surgeon would prefer to hear from you sooner rather than later)

This list doesn't include everything you may possibly encounter — no list could. So, if you feel concerned about *anything* you're feeling, call your surgeon. You're better off calling and finding out that it's nothing to worry about than not calling and having the problem get worse. Yes, your doctor will tell you to come in to be checked out. Better to be checked out and have nothing wrong or discover something early than let something brew for a while that will put you in danger. Communication with your surgeon is very important for the rest of your life — and it's especially critical in the first few weeks after surgery.

Before your surgery, discuss with your surgeon which hospital to go to in case of emergency. Unless you live very near where you had your weight loss surgery, you may not be able to travel to that hospital if you experience problems. Some hospitals will be better than others at dealing with the kinds of problems you may encounter. Your surgeon will be best able to advise you.

Getting the Help You Need

When you return home after surgery, you've definitely made progress, but you still have some more recovering to do. You won't be able to resume your normal routine or pace right away, and that means you may need some help. In the following sections, we give you some suggestions for finding help with your kids and your household responsibilities, and we also fill you in on some issues to consider if you live by yourself.

Caring for your kids

Your kids may see your surgery as a one-day event. They may not realize that you have a lot of healing to do after your surgery, both mentally and physically. Little ones will wave their arms and want to be picked up, and teenagers will want you to care for and cater to them just as you did before.

You can make your recovery time much smoother for everyone involved if you talk to your kids ahead of time about what they can expect when you get home from the hospital. If they know what's coming, they'll be better able to handle it — even if they need a reminder now and then.

Your kids need to understand that you'll have some limitations in the first few weeks after your surgery. Your surgeon will probably warn you that you can't lift more than 10 to 15 pounds for the first four to six weeks. That means no lifting children, laundry baskets, or other things you're used to picking up.

In a year, you'll be much healthier and probably weight-lifting that much or more! But for the time being, take it easy.

If possible, ask a family member or close friend to stay with you after your surgery — even if you have a spouse or partner and especially if you have younger children. An extra set of hands around the house to help out with the kids will put your mind at ease. If you're very weak and unable to do much, you'll be very happy that you asked for help. If you feel fine, you can always cancel or just sit back and enjoy some pampering for a few days.

Between the pampering and the naps, you still need to walk, walk, walk.

You may want to tap into some other sources of help when it comes to your kids. For example, you can use babysitters even when you're home. Neighborhood middle-school students can be the perfect age. They're a little too young to leave alone with small children, but they're great for when you're in the house recovering from surgery. You'll be available to answer questions and help in an emergency, but they'll be doing most of the work and playing with your little ones. Plus, they'll probably be less expensive than older kids — and more available. And they'll also probably love the chance to get some babysitting experience under their belts. If you have kids who are a little older and more involved in after-school activities, you may want to recruit some neighborhood high-school students. They can take on more responsibility than their middle-school counterparts.

Parents of your children's friends are another great resource. You know your children will be content if they're playing at their friends' houses. Ask if your kids can spend some extra time there after school for a few days until you're better able to take care of them yourself. Offer to return the favor after you have your energy back.

Keeping house

Weight loss surgery is major surgery, and most patients have some health issues going into the surgery, so they aren't in tip-top shape to begin with. When you return home, healing is your number-one priority. But life does go on, and certain things around the house do demand your attention. How will you handle them?

Start by following some of the advice we give in Chapter 8 and preparing ahead of time by lining up the help you need.

You also may want to call a cleaning service and have someone else take care of your housecleaning for two or three weeks after surgery. This way, you won't have to look at the mess.

In addition, talk to your spouse or partner about anything you would like him or her to do in the first few weeks after you get home from the hospital. If your spouse or partner is prepared by knowing ahead of time what you need, things may go more smoothly. Don't expect anyone to read your mind. Talk about what kind of help you'll need around the house, and if your spouse or partner won't be able to pick up the slack, you can plan ahead of time to get some outside help.

Think about how you'll handle mealtimes. Cooking meals ahead of time and freezing them works well. That way, all you (or your spouse or kids) have to do is pop something in the microwave.

It won't kill your family not to have the sheets changed your first week home, or not to have fresh towels during your healing time. If the house is a disaster for a little while, it's not the end of the world. If you're naturally a perfectionist, the idea of a house that Martha Stewart wouldn't want to call her own may drive you crazy. But while you're healing, try to lighten up and let it slide. You'll have much more energy after you start losing weight, and you can use it to catch up on some of the housework that you had to put on the back burner while you recuperated.

Looking out for yourself if you live alone

Having weight loss surgery is difficult enough when you have people at home to support you. It can bring particular challenges if you're coming home by yourself. Don't try doing it all. Look for as many sources of help as you can.

As we mention in Chapter 9, see if you can be discharged to the rehab department in the hospital, instead of going straight home. If your surgeon determines that being on your own isn't safe, you may be able to get your stay in rehab covered by your insurance. Though you're probably eager to get out of the hospital, you'll be steadier and better able to take care of yourself after working on your mobility and strength in rehab.

Whether you can get into the rehab center after your surgery or you end up going straight home, talk with friends and neighbors and ask for the help you need. Being self-sufficient is a wonderful thing, but when you're recovering from major surgery, you need a helping hand. Don't allow your pride to stand in the way of your getting the help you need.

Here are some other things you may consider:

- **Take advantage of a home health service.** There are home health services that will stay with you for a four-hour minimum per day. They'll probably be covered by your insurance if you need them for medical reasons.

- **Check out your surgeon's support group.** It may have an "angel" committee — former patients who volunteer to help those who've just had surgery. Most often, they just visit in the hospital and are available for phone consultations, but you may want to see if anyone would be willing to spend a few hours with you for a few days. This is another excellent reason to attend the support group prior to surgery — the support group meetings are where you can meet these people and put in your request.

- **If you have a good friend with a spare bedroom, you may find it best to move in with that friend for a few days.** This may even be more convenient for your friend than having to frequently pop in and check on you. If you're right there, you can get help when you need it, and your friend may worry less about you.

Keeping Up with Your Meds

Before your surgery, you were probably already taking some medications to address some of your health issues. But after your surgery, your body changes very rapidly — and so do your body's needs.

Some patients leave the hospital not needing many of their medications. Others still need the same medications, but in different dosages. Whatever your situation, be sure to follow your doctor's instructions exactly.

A little too much togetherness!

Many couples decide that they both want to have weight loss surgery and question the when and how. Going through the surgery at the same time may seem like a good idea — you may like the thought of sharing the experience, along with the highs and lows. But having weight loss surgery at the same time as your spouse or partner is a bad idea. If you have your surgeries at the same time, you won't be able to support one another very well. Plus, any problems you have will be multiplied. And you may even find yourself competing with one another in your weight loss, or resenting one another if the other person appears to have it easier.

We recommend spacing your surgeries at least six weeks apart. That way, the first person to have the surgery will have completely recovered and be prepared to assist the second person when it's his or her turn.

If you have trouble swallowing pills

If you have to take medication after your surgery, and you're at all concerned about swallowing them, here are some tips:

✔ **If your medication is the size of a Tic Tac or smaller, try swallowing your pill and see what happens.** You may have less trouble than you expect. If the pill does get stuck in your throat, it will be very uncomfortable, but it will eventually dissolve. Try taking some big gulps of water to get the pill to go down.

✔ **Buy a pill splitter and cut your pills in half or in pieces.** You can find a pill splitter at your local pharmacy. Sometimes just reducing the size of really large pills is enough to help you swallow them without any trouble.

✔ **Crush them and mix them with a little bit of juice or applesauce (if you're allowed to eat it).** If splitting the pills doesn't do the trick, try crushing the medication and taking it in juice or something soft (as long as you have the green light to eat).

✔ **If the pill is a capsule, open it.** It may not taste so good, but if you can't swallow pills because of your surgery, this is the best option.

✔ **Ask your doctor or pharmacist if your medication comes in a liquid form, can be crushed, or comes in a capsule that can be opened.**

✔ **Buy all vitamins and supplements in a chewable or liquid form, especially the first few months after surgery.**

Check with your doctor about taking time-release pills. Time-release pills are not absorbed in the same way as non-time-release pills, so they may have a different effect after gastric bypass surgery. (This doesn't apply after gastric banding surgery or sleeve gastrectomy.) You also may want to check with the consumer affairs department of the drug company that manufactures your medication to see if it has any information regarding its drug and gastric bypass patients. (Many prescribing physicians are not experts on the absorption of medications following gastric bypass surgery, so you may have to do a little research of your own.)

Coordinating your meds with your doctor

With rapid weight loss, many patients experience a rapid improvement in their overall health. You may not need the same medications you needed before your surgery, and the medications and dosages you do need may be in flux for a while as you go through the adjustment of losing a large amount of weight.

Follow the advice of your doctor very carefully. Even though other patients may not need their medication after surgery, don't jeopardize your health by being hasty. Your doctor will determine your needs.

Make sure you maintain good communication with your doctor so she's familiar with your weight loss and watching for any changes required with your medications. Otherwise, you may end up being overmedicated and experience some negative side effects.

Knowing which over-the-counter meds are okay and which you should avoid

In general, taking non-steroidal anti-inflammatory drugs (NSAIDs) after weight loss surgery is not a good idea. NSAIDs (such as aspirin, Advil, and Aleve) can cause bleeding and ulcers. You have to stay off NSAIDS for one to two weeks after surgery. If you need to take NSAIDs after these two weeks, let your surgeon know and ask for guidelines about how much you can take.

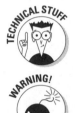

After both gastric bypass surgery and gastric banding surgery, the surface area of the new pouch is very small. When you take an NSAID, it will likely fall on or near the same spot every time. Therefore, the chance of bleeding and ulcers is increased.

Tylenol (acetaminophen) is okay to take. But here are some over-the-counter meds you should avoid:

- ✔ Advil
- ✔ Aleve
- ✔ Alka-Seltzer
- ✔ Aspirin
- ✔ Bufferin
- ✔ Coricidin
- ✔ Cortisone
- ✔ Excedrin
- ✔ Fiorinol
- ✔ Ibuprofen
- ✔ Motrin
- ✔ Vanquish

If you have any questions about which medications you can take after your weight loss surgery, check with your surgeon.

If you have to take aspirin for your heart, clear it with your surgeon and then take a chewable form so it doesn't sit in your new stomach.

Recognizing the Signs of Depression

The few weeks right after surgery are often really difficult. When you're in pain and still recuperating, you may find yourself wondering what you've done to your body and why. You may have nausea and have trouble keeping even liquids down. You can easily start to think that your life will always be like this — seeing beyond this period of recovery is often difficult.

In the weeks following surgery, you need to look to your support systems and focus on the positive. You made it through the surgery, and you've started losing weight! You can breathe better, and you may be able to move better. You're on the road to recovery, and if you hadn't had the courage to go forward with your weight loss surgery, your life wouldn't have been changing for the better.

If something really has you down, call your surgeon or one of the staff in the surgeon's office to get the help you need. Here's a list of some common symptoms of depression following weight loss surgery. If you experience one or more of these symptoms, call your surgeon and discuss some possible treatment options:

- A feeling of sadness that just won't go away
- A feeling that everything is hopeless
- A feeling that you're worthless and helpless
- A total disinterest in things that interested you before
- Thoughts of death or suicide
- The inability to sleep or the inability to stay awake
- Being restless or irritable

For more information on depression, go to the website of the National Institute of Mental Health (www.nimh.nih.gov/health/publications/depression/complete-index.shtml) and call the office of your surgeon. Healthcare professionals affiliated with your surgeon will be able to help you.

Turn to Chapter 19 for even more information on depression following weight loss surgery.

The road ahead for the next few months won't be easy, but rest assured that life *will* get better. The feelings you have now are a small price to pay for a future life of good health.

Chapter 13

Hi-Ho, Hi-Ho, It's Back to Work You Go!

In This Chapter

▶ Identifying the factors that affect your readiness

▶ Making sure you don't rush your return

▶ Responding to your co-workers

Returning to work is one of the last steps you'll take toward getting your life back to normal — or at least reestablishing some of the daily routines that were part of your life before your surgery. Whether you're champing at the bit, eager to return to work, or you're dreading the return and the questions you're sure you'll face from your co-workers, you need to know when the time is right. Returning to work before your body is ready will only slow your recovery — and it may even bring about a setback you wouldn't have faced otherwise.

In this chapter, we help you determine when you're ready to return to work. We also prepare you for some of your co-workers' reactions to your surgery — from supportive to negative and everything in between. Finally, we help you figure out how much to tell your co-workers and how much to keep to yourself.

Knowing Whether You're Ready to Punch the Clock

The amount of time you'll need at home to recover from your surgery is unique to your body and your situation — and it depends on many factors. Some people need as little as two weeks to recover; others need six weeks or more. Although you may know someone who went back to work very soon after weight loss surgery, the important thing is to return when *you* have had enough recovery time.

If you need more recovery time than someone else, that doesn't mean there's something wrong with you. Each person recovers from surgery at his or her own rate. Everything from how fast you lose weight to how soon you progress to certain foods to how soon you go back to work is unique to you — there's no right or wrong about it.

In the following sections, we help you identify some of the factors that will contribute to how long you'll need to recover before going back to work, and we help you figure out whether you're ready.

Being aware of the factors that affect how ready you are

Your ability to return to work will be impacted by several key factors, including the following:

- ✔ **The kind of surgery you had:** If you had gastric banding surgery, you'll be able to go back to work sooner than if you had gastric bypass, sleeve gastrectomy, or duodenal switch surgery. Gastric banding patients typically go back to work in one or two weeks. Gastric bypass, sleeve gastrectomy, and duodenal switch patients generally go back to work in two to four weeks.

- ✔ **Whether you had surgery done as an open incision or laparoscopically:** If the surgery was done open, you may need more time to recover than if your surgery was done laparoscopically.

- ✔ **Whether you had health challenges before surgery or complications during surgery:** If you had any complications during surgery or if you had many health challenges prior to surgery, you may need more time to recover.

- ✔ **The kind of work you do:** If you have a desk job or a job that doesn't require much physical activity, you may be able to return to work sooner than if your job is more physically demanding.

- ✔ **Your company rules:** If your company allows employees to return part-time, you'll be able to return to work sooner. Some businesses see employees returning on a limited basis as a liability — they see it as an indication that you aren't completely healed, and they may require you to wait until you can comfortably work a full day before you return. *Remember:* Find out your company's rules before your surgery, so you know what to expect during your recovery.

Making sure you're ready

You may be anxious to get back to work, but don't rush it. Always follow the advice of your doctor — if your surgeon says you aren't ready yet, you're better off waiting a while longer. If you try to return too soon, it may harm your recovery.

Here are some questions to ask yourself to help you figure out if you're ready to return to work:

- **Do you still require frequent naps or rests during the day?** If so, you aren't ready. You won't be able to stop when you need to at work.

- **Are you sleeping well at night?** Because of your incisions, some people need a while before they can rest comfortably. Poor sleeping will mean you'll be even more tired during working hours.

- **Are you still on pain medication?** If so, you won't be thinking clearly enough for work.

- **Have you figured out that you need to take small sips throughout the day to get in 64 ounces of noncaloric fluids?** When you go back to your work routine, this may be harder to do, so get it under your belt before you go back. Think about taking in 4 ounces (½ cup) every hour!

- **Has your doctor given you the thumbs-up?** If your doctor says you're ready, you are. If your doctor doesn't think your body is up for it just yet, be patient and wait a little longer. Your body will thank you for it.

Whenever you do return to work, keep in mind that your first week will be extremely tiring. At home, you had the luxury of resting or napping whenever you felt the need. On the job, you'll have to tough it out.

Anticipating Your Co-workers' Responses to Your Surgery

You probably spend at least as much time with your colleagues as you do with your family. Yet your co-workers most likely haven't had the advantage of an orientation to weight loss surgery. They're approaching your return to work with their own knowledge — or lack of it — and with their own misconceptions and maybe even prejudices.

Some of your co-workers may be incredibly supportive and welcoming when you return. Others may be glad to see you but a little unsure how to behave when you're around. And others may see your return as their cue to offer up their not-so-positive opinions on weight loss surgery.

Educating your colleagues about your surgery and the aftereffects you're anticipating *before* you go into the hospital can be a huge help. Explain why you're taking such a drastic step, so they'll better understand what you're going through when you return.

Weight loss surgery: No one's idea of a vacation

Many people decide to use their limited vacation days for their surgery recovery. If you do that, you may find yourself pushing to return to work sooner rather than later. When your vacation time is up, you'll have to go back regardless of how you feel.

Using a short amount of vacation time to recover from your weight loss surgery is dangerous because you'll be inclined to have the vacation days — not your health — dictate your return. You want to make sure that, when you return to work, it's because your body is truly ready — not because you've used up all the vacation time you had saved up. And we don't have to tell you that weight loss surgery is *not* a vacation.

Before your surgery, talk to your employer and see if you can arrange for any other ways to allow for your recovery time, and plan for the possibility that you may need more time than you think. Stress that in the long run your overall health will improve, and along with it your absenteeism and productivity will improve as well. Here are some possibilities to consider:

✔ **Take some time without pay.** If possible, try to sock away some extra money (living expenses for a month or two) in case you need to take some time off without pay. If

you end up not needing it, you can keep that money as a nice little nest egg, or use it to reward yourself with a dream vacation after you've lost the weight and improved your health.

✔ **Find out if you can do some work at home.** As your recovery progresses, you may be able to do some work for an hour or two here or there throughout the day, resting and taking naps when you need to. If you have access to your work e-mail at home, you may be able to ease back into work slowly, which not only helps your employer (who reaps the reward of your work) but also helps you feel less overwhelmed when you actually do return to the office. Just make sure to go at your own pace and don't take on more than you're ready for — whether you're working from home or going back to work full-time.

✔ **See if you can be put on administrative duties or light duty for a short time.** Depending on your job, if you're able to have your daily responsibilities reduced a bit when you first return, you may be able to get back to work a little earlier than you would otherwise. Plus, the transition back may be an easier one.

In the following sections, we help you respond to your co-workers — no matter how they respond to you.

Answering (or not answering) your co-workers' questions

When you return to work, one of two things will happen: Either you'll face a barrage of questions from your co-workers, or they'll be afraid to ask you what they're really wondering. How you respond to your co-workers' natural curiosity depends on your personality and how private you are. If you're naturally gregarious and your life is an open book, you may have no problem holding forth at the water cooler on the nitty-gritty details of your surgery. If you're on the shy side, or you just don't think it's anybody's business, you may prefer to keep your surgery to yourself.

There is no right or wrong way to respond to your co-workers. What's important is that you prepare for their reactions before you return, so you have a strategy for responding — whatever that strategy may be.

Be prepared for people to ask you anything and everything about weight loss surgery. Most people are very curious about it, and they may come right out and ask — whether you want them to or not.

Be equally prepared for people to watch everything you put in your mouth. Your diet will be a great curiosity for many of your colleagues. People will want to know what you're eating and whether you feel hungry. Some people may admonish you every time they see you eat something — believe it or not, they may even think that their interference is helpful. You may hear, "Should you be eating that?" when you're eating something that's perfectly acceptable on your post-surgery diet. Try to plan for how you'll respond if someone asks you a question like this. If you know how you'll respond, you'll be less likely to be rattled when the question arises.

If you're a private person, you may not want to tell *anyone* why you were off work for a few weeks. You may be embarrassed that you needed surgery to get control of your weight. You may not want to deal with all the questions! And you may be unsure that you'll really be successful following the surgery. Of course, deciding whether to tell your co-workers about your surgery — and how much to tell them — is your call.

If you're tempted to explain away your weight loss to dieting and exercise, keep in mind that you'll be losing weight so rapidly that people will want to know your secret. And there may be times when you're out with your co-workers and you'll either eat something that doesn't agree with you or you won't chew it well enough and up that food will come. If you really don't want to let people know your business, you need to be prepared for some of these situations and do what you can to prevent or at least manage them.

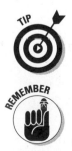

If you're concerned about eating in front of clients, plan on having soup or some soft fish. This strategy is especially important in the early months after surgery. Plan ahead and check out menus so you know your options. Forewarned is forearmed!

Colleagues, customers, or clients you see only once or twice a year probably won't recognize you the next time they see you. They may ask what's happened to you. Or they may be hesitant to ask, and you may wonder if they've even noticed your weight loss. Chances are, they've noticed, but they're just too shy to ask. If you're comfortable doing so, tell them about it upfront; doing so can make your relationships a lot more comfortable and put their minds at ease.

The easy way out? Hardly!

Nothing is more infuriating to someone who has had weight loss surgery than being accused of taking "the easy way out." You know what you've been through. You've tried dieting and failed over and over. You've probably struggled to get insurance coverage, been frightened about dying during surgery, and endured pain and nausea afterward. So, understandably, you have little patience with someone who characterizes what you've been through as "easy"!

If you're faced with someone — whether at work or elsewhere — who doesn't hesitate to tell you that you've taken the easy way out, you have two choices: You can ignore him or

enlighten him. If you ignore him, he'll continue to have this misconception — but you'll be spared the debate. If you enlighten him, he may have a better appreciation for why you've gone through this surgery and what you've been through.

If you can't explain everything sufficiently, give him a copy of this book. And realize that you may just have to agree to disagree on this topic. You can't convince everybody that weight loss surgery isn't an easy way out. But you also can't allow people who don't understand to affect the way you feel about yourself or your decision.

Avoiding being left out

After surgery, you undergo some pretty rapid changes, and your colleagues may react to those changes in ways you don't expect. For example, before your surgery, you may have gone out to lunch with the gang every Friday. After your surgery, you may find that you're being left out of those regular get-togethers.

If this sounds familiar, it's possible that your colleagues are uncomfortable eating around you. They may think that they're tempting you to eat when you've gone to such drastic measures *not* to eat. They may prefer not adding to your stress or not putting themselves under stress when all they want to do is enjoy a relaxing lunch.

Many people also are under the odd impression that weight loss surgery patients just don't eat — at all! They may think that part of your life — eating — has been left behind. They don't realize that you *do* eat — you just eat small portions.

You also may be left out of office birthday celebrations because your co-workers won't know how you'll handle eating cake. People are culturally accustomed to having everything center around food, and your colleagues may not realize that you'd love to join in the celebration and just pass up the cake.

If you're being left out, speak up and let your friends know that you still want to be part of the lunches and parties. They may not know what to do, and your mentioning it will probably relieve them.

Dodging resentments

Most of your colleagues will cheer your efforts to tackle your weight problems. They'll realize the tremendous courage and determination that you had
in order to take such a major step. But a few people may resent you. Here are
some reasons behind that resentment:

- **If someone in your office has had to pick up the slack while you were
  off, she may hold it against you.** This will be especially true if she
  thinks your surgery was cosmetic and the only reason that you're the
  way you are is because you're lazy and lack self-control. She'll see your
  time away as an unnecessary cause of her having to work overtime.

  If you suspect this may be the case, speak with your co-worker about
  the importance of weight loss to control many health problems. Tell her
  how you repeatedly tried other measures and this was your only hope
  to control your weight. And thank her for everything she did to help out
  while you were away. Sometimes all people need is to feel appreciated. A
  simple "thank you" — or a note or even a small gift — can go a long way
  toward ridding your office of resentment.

- **As you lose weight, you'll no longer be the largest person in the office,
  and the person who's now the largest may resent you for that.** He may
  have known he was heavy, but at least he wasn't as heavy as you. With
  your recent weight loss, he may now have to face his own obesity — and
  he may very well take that out on you. If you think this may be the case,
  you can't really do much to control the situation. Just do your best to
  understand that this has nothing to do with you and everything to do
  with the person's own feelings about himself. Be as kind as you can be,
  and try to remember what it felt like to be in that person's shoes.

- **Some colleagues may resent the way you're changing in nonphysical
  ways.** You're a different person following surgery, and people don't
  always react favorably to change. Many people find that, before their
  surgery, they may have let people take advantage of them, but after their
  surgery, as they lose weight and gain self-esteem, they're less inclined
  to be anybody's doormat. Your personality may change along with your
  tolerance. Your increasing independence may be a source of someone
  else's stress. Your newfound confidence may cause a little friction, especially if you're asserting yourself for the first time. Recognize that this is
  just part of the territory, and know that, in time, your colleagues will get
  to know — and like — the new you just as they did the old one.

Part IV

This Time I'm Going to Make It: Ensuring Success

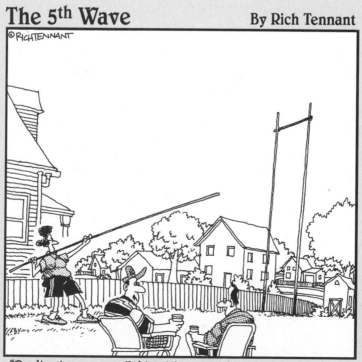

The 5th Wave   By Rich Tennant

"Don't get me wrong. I think it's great that Barbara decided she wanted to start exercising more after her surgery."

In this part . . .

How do you define success? It isn't just the number on your bathroom scale — it's also the condition of your health and the quality of your life. In this part, we look at expectations and what happens when they are or aren't met.

Here, you also discover what it takes to be successful and healthy in the long term. We outline eating patterns, exercises, and nutritional supplements that will keep you in good shape for a lifetime.

And you don't have to go it alone: There are support groups to tap into, made up of people who have gone through exactly what you're experiencing — they're invaluable for nonmedical advice and commiseration.

Chapter 14

What Is Success Anyway?

*B*efore your weight loss surgery, you probably spent a lot of time focused on the surgery and recovery — you were caught up in figuring out whether the surgery was right for you, seeing whether your insurance company would cover it, finding the best surgeon, and getting back into the routines of daily life after the surgery. Losing weight and improving your health were your goals, and you had your eyes set on that.

But months after your surgery, you may be a little unsure whether you've met your goal. If you're not yet at your ideal weight, does that mean you're a success or a failure? What does it mean to succeed?

In this chapter, we take a look at what makes a success and give you an opportunity to define success for yourself, using measures other than just weight loss.

Defining Success

When it comes to weight loss surgery, different people have differing views of success. Although *you* may not consider yourself a success until you've lost 100 percent of your excess weight, your surgeon has an entirely different view.

With conventional dieting alone (and no surgery), the medical profession would consider you a success if you maintained a 5 percent weight loss. With weight loss surgery, you'll lose a much greater percentage than that — so you've already made great progress.

ANECDOTE

My most cherished success

My life has changed in so many wondrous and unexpected ways. I feel no shame when looking into a mirror, I have no frustration in trying to find cute clothes that will fit, and I have no embarrassment when trying to fit into restaurant and airplane seats. The dark cloud that hung over my head, which represented the pain and shame, has completely vanished. I truly walk in sunshine each and every day; there are no more obstacles.

When people ask me what is the best and worst thing about this surgery, I honestly tell them that it's knowing there is nothing I cannot accomplish. Physical limitations certainly went away, and my mental and spiritual outlook on life also got a tremendous boost — for the first time in my life, I am in control! The thought of growing old with my husband was never a realistic goal, and now it will be my most cherished success.

Teesha Murphy
Thornton, Colorado

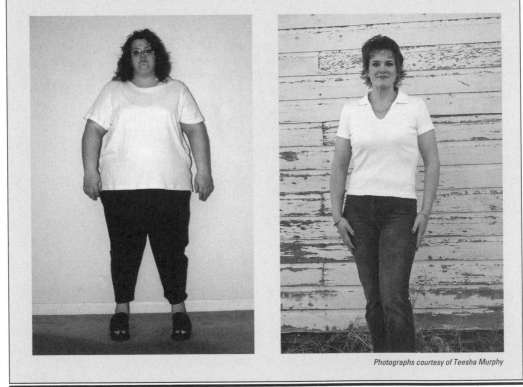

Photographs courtesy of Teesha Murphy

REMEMBER

That said, in all likelihood, you probably won't lose 100 percent of your excess weight and keep it off forever. In fact, surgeons consider you successful if you're able to lose 50 percent of your excess weight and keep it off for five years or more.

Keeping Your Expectations Real

Be clear about what you want and what you can expect from your weight loss surgery. **Remember:** The operation is not a magic pill. It works with you, not around you. Your commitment to a healthy lifestyle, which includes a healthy diet and increased activity, is crucial.

Weight loss is a lot like taking a test. At first, you hope you passed, and when you do, you wish you'd done better. Likewise, most patients have a weight loss goal in mind, and when they get near it, they lower that goal by another 20 to 30 pounds.

Modifying your goals isn't necessarily a bad thing to do — but you do need to keep in mind that none of the weight loss surgeries allow the average patient to get to the ideal body weight. With diet and exercise, you certainly *can* get to your ideal body weight after surgery, but your weight loss surgery only takes you so far — the rest you have to do yourself (with diet and exercise).

Instead of using a magic number (like the weight you were in high school, or the weight you were when you got married) as your goal, keep in mind the range of weights that are healthy by using the body mass index (BMI) chart in Table 14-1. Just as you used BMI to determine whether you were qualified to have weight loss surgery (in Chapter 2), you can use the BMI chart to determine whether you've achieved a realistic (and healthy!) goal weight.

A BMI of 25 to 29.9 is considered overweight, and a BMI of 30 to 39.9 is considered obese. (Turn to Chapter 2 for more information on BMI.) On average, weight loss surgery will bring you to a BMI in the range of 25 to 35 depending on your starting BMI.

If your goal is a BMI below 24.9 but above 19.9 that means your weight is in the "normal" range. But if you don't reach that "normal" range, don't feel that you're a failure. Being in the "overweight" range is far better than being in the "severely obese" range. Give yourself credit for your wonderful success!

Anything lower than 18.5 is considered underweight; if you have a BMI that puts you in the underweight category, make an appointment with your surgeon so you can discuss the possible reasons and get your weight back into the healthy range. **Remember:** Being underweight can be just as dangerous as being overweight.

Table 14-1

Body Mass Index

Height (inches)	Body Weight (pounds)																
BMI	19	20	21	22	23	24	25	26	27	28	29	30	31	32	33	34	35
58	91	96	100	105	110	115	119	124	129	134	138	143	148	153	158	162	167
59	94	99	104	109	114	119	124	128	133	138	143	148	153	158	163	168	173
60	97	102	107	112	118	123	128	133	138	143	148	153	158	163	168	174	179
61	100	106	111	116	122	127	132	137	143	148	153	158	164	169	174	180	185
62	104	109	115	120	126	131	136	142	147	153	158	164	169	175	180	186	191
63	107	113	118	124	130	135	141	146	152	158	163	169	174	180	186	191	197
64	110	116	122	128	134	140	145	151	157	163	169	174	180	186	192	197	204
65	114	120	126	132	138	144	150	156	162	168	174	180	186	192	198	204	210
66	118	124	130	136	142	148	155	161	167	173	179	186	192	198	204	210	216
67	121	127	134	140	146	153	159	166	172	178	185	191	198	204	211	217	223
68	125	131	138	144	151	158	164	171	177	184	190	197	203	210	216	223	230
69	128	135	142	149	155	162	169	176	182	189	196	203	209	216	223	230	236
70	132	139	146	153	160	167	174	181	188	195	202	209	216	222	229	236	243
71	136	143	150	157	165	172	179	186	193	200	208	215	222	229	236	243	250
72	140	147	154	162	169	177	184	191	199	206	213	221	228	235	242	250	258
73	144	151	159	166	174	182	189	197	204	212	219	227	235	242	250	257	265
74	148	155	163	171	179	186	194	202	210	218	225	233	241	249	256	264	272
75	152	160	168	176	184	192	200	208	216	224	232	240	248	256	264	272	279
76	156	164	172	180	189	197	205	213	221	230	238	246	254	263	271	279	287

ANECDOTE

Two days before surgery . . .

Two days before surgery and all through the house, not a creature was stirring, not even a mouse, but I was going crazy and nervous as could be, because in two short days, there would be a new me.

The hardest time for me was the two days before surgery. I had been eating to my heart's content everything I could, because I knew that in a short period of time, I wouldn't be able to gorge myself like I had in the past.

I was just sick and tired of food. Can you believe that, coming from a man of 396 pounds? I had eaten myself into a frenzy, and then the brakes were put on two days before surgery, when I was limited to soft foods like pudding, mashed potatoes, clear soups, and clear drinks.

I admit that my brain was playing games with me — it was telling me that this wouldn't keep my old body alive, and that I needed more. I got the headaches, felt faint, and lost all my energy. I thought I was going to die from starvation.

One day before surgery, I was on clear liquids. I was so hungry and weak that I didn't think I would make it to surgery the next day.

Surgery day came, and I was nervous. I didn't think about being hungry any longer. Dr. Rose Marie Jones came in for a visit before I walked back for surgery and said that I wouldn't wake up hungry! She was right.

I am now at 212 pounds and I have to admit that I haven't been hungry since. My recommendation to people about to have weight loss surgery: Work or at least keep busy for those two days before surgery. Keep your mind busy so you don't have to think about what you're not eating or what you are eating.

I just wish I had done the surgery much sooner. I'm off all my medications. I have an amazing amount of energy. I'm a new person because of a tool given to me to help me control my obesity.

Tony Augsburger

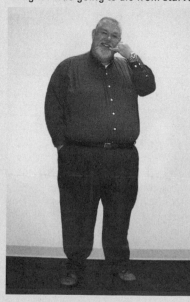 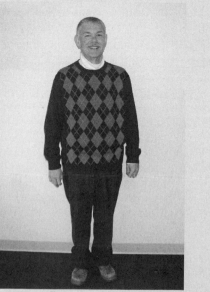

Photographs courtesy of Tony Augsburger

Seizing the Window of Opportunity

The *window of opportunity* is that period of time after surgery when losing weight is easiest. The weight may just seem to come off without effort — you're in weight-loss heaven! Sure, you may hit a plateau now and then, but these are minor setbacks on what seems to be a dream journey to your ideal weight. Or, you may have to struggle harder, but the weight still comes off.

When your weight loss slows, that's a sign that the window of opportunity is closing. This window usually closes at the end of the first year for gastric bypass patients. Because the gastric banding is adjustable and the duodenal switch is so malabsorptive, patients continue to lose at a slower rate during the second year.

The window of opportunity closes for a variety of reasons:

 ✔ **As you lose weight, you burn fewer calories.** For example, if you weigh 125 pounds and walk for 10 minutes, you burn 44 calories. If you weigh 200 pounds and walk that same 10 minutes, you burn 70 calories.

 ✔ **With gastric bypass and sleeve gastrectomy surgery, your new stomach may stretch a little, which will allow you to eat more food. Also, in gastric bypass surgery, your *stoma* (the opening to your small intestine) may stretch.** That means food won't remain in your pouch but will empty too soon into your intestines. The bottom line: You'll get hungry faster and end up eating more.

 ✔ **With gastric bypass and duodenal switch surgeries, your body will adjust a bit to the malabsorption, and you'll absorb more calories than you did immediately after surgery.**

 ✔ **When you look good and feel good, having the motivation to work hard at losing those last few pounds may be difficult.**

Although the fastest weight loss occurs within the first year, you can still continue losing weight, depending on what you do with your diet and how active you are.

Most weight loss surgery patients start a maintenance program at a year, and what some people do for maintenance actually contributes to further weight loss. *Maintenance* means you're figuring out what to eat and how active to be in order to maintain your weight. You should do this in conjunction with the dietitian associated with your surgeon's practice.

Never forget that losing weight is a constant battle. You'll battle the head hunger and food demons for the rest of your life. Chapter 15 provides you with tips on eating strategies you can use forever.

Make sure your goal weight is *your* goal (not anybody else's) and discuss it with your surgeon to make sure that goal is attainable. Don't let someone else tell you that you're too skinny or too fat. Weight loss surgery can empower you and improve your self-esteem. Let it also allow you to determine where your weight should be.

Looking At Successes Beyond Weight Loss

Part of your goal in having weight loss surgery was to lose weight, but you also had weight loss surgery to correct your obesity-related health problems. Because of that, some surgeons like to measure a patient's success by how it improves those health conditions, instead of just by weight loss alone.

For example, let's say you had diabetes and you were 100 pounds over-weight. After your surgery, you lost 45 pounds (so 45 percent of your excess weight) and you were no longer diabetic. Would you be a success or a fail-ure? Based on the weight loss criteria alone, you haven't lost 50 percent of your excess weight. But the surgery cured your diabetes, so some surgeons would say the surgery was successful.

The following is a list of some of the obesity-related health problems that can be cured or reduced after weight loss surgery. If you've seen improvement or cure of these conditions, you also may be able to consider your surgery a success, whether you've lost 50 percent of your excess weight or not. (If you have questions about this issue, as always, talk with your surgeon.)

- ✔ **Diabetes:** With duodenal switch, sleeve gastrectomy, and gastric bypass surgeries, type 2 diabetes can be cured or improved 80 percent to 100 percent of the time. With gastric banding, type 2 diabetes can be cured or improved 70 percent to 90 percent of the time. The results for patients with type 1 diabetes vary a bit more, but improvements are still common.

- ✔ **Hypertension (high blood pressure):** With sustained weight loss, high blood pressure can improve or be cured in up to 85 percent of patients with gastric bypass, sleeve gastrectomy, and duodenal switch surgeries and in up to 70 percent of patients with gastric banding. Your doctor may still want you on some heart-protective medications, so follow-up with your primary-care physician is crucial.

- ✔ **Obstructive sleep apnea:** Sleep apnea can be *obstructive* (meaning that the soft tissues in your throat block your air passage when you sleep) or *central* (meaning that your breathing pattern stems from the brain). Weight loss surgery helps improve or cure sleep apnea only if it's obstructive. So, if you have central sleep apnea or a mixed type of sleep apnea (with elements of both), only the obstructive pattern can be improved or resolved. Obstructive sleep apnea improves with as little as 10 percent of total body weight loss (so if you weighed 300 pounds going into the surgery, if you lose just 30 pounds, your obstructive sleep apnea is improved).

- **Osteoarthritis (joint pain):** Not all joint pain is osteoarthritis. Osteoarthritis is bone-on-bone pain and inflammation due to degeneration within the joint, and it's one of the health problems related to severe obesity. Weight loss can significantly improve joint pain — when you lose 10 pounds, it's like taking 30 to 40 pounds off your knees! The degeneration that is within the joint doesn't improve, but it progresses at a slower rate (that is, it continues to get worse, just not as quickly as it would have if you hadn't lost weight).

- **Asthma:** Asthma can worsen with severe obesity, and it improves with sustained weight loss. Asthmatics have *reactive airways* (meaning that your airway can narrow with cold, stress, and other triggers, and cause wheezing), and even with weight loss they continue to have reactive airways. The airways of asthmatics just react less after they've lost a significant amount of weight. This means fewer admissions to the hospital and fewer treatments with heavy-duty asthma medications like steroids.

- **Gastroesophageal reflux disease (GERD):** Reflux of acid into the esophagus occurs fairly often in those who are severely obese. With weight loss, the reflux symptoms improve or disappear completely. After gastric bypass surgery, the pouch is so small, and the contents usually empty so quickly into the intestine, that there isn't much that can reflux back into the esophagus. With gastric banding, the band acts as a barrier to prevent the stomach contents from refluxing into the esophagus. Occasionally, band patients experience heartburn after they eat, but this is usually related to food sliding back and forth in the esophagus, which is food regurgitation. In sleeve gastrectomy, duodenal switch, and biliopancreatic diversion patients, reflux can still occur because the gastric pouch is larger — but the symptoms overall may still improve with weight loss. Hiatal hernia repair is becoming more common at the time of weight loss surgery and will decrease the likelihood of experiencing GERD symptoms.

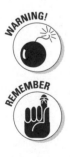

Not all cases of diabetes, high blood pressure, and sleep apnea are cured. If you have these disorders, close follow-up with your primary-care doctor and your surgeon is very important.

Even though you'll likely notice a tremendous improvement in how you feel after weight loss surgery, you may have some conditions that won't improve with weight loss:

- **Back pain and herniated discs:** Back pain and pain related to herniated discs may improve with weight loss, but these problems are seldom cured. Herniated discs don't slip back into place despite weight loss. At best, pain is improved or made more manageable because you're carrying less weight. Weight loss may make you a better candidate for procedures that can help your back pain, though.

✔ **Thyroid disease:** Thyroid disease is not a health problem directly caused by severe obesity but, interestingly, some patients who take the medication Synthroid require less of this medication with sustained weight loss.

After you've lost a significant amount of weight, you may feel more energetic and years younger. You may feel as though you've recaptured some of your youth or the youth that you should have had but didn't because of your severe obesity.

But some days, expect to feel a little depressed and wish that you could turn back the clock to when you could self-medicate with food. Thankfully, those days are few and far between as you lead a more active and healthy life.

Enjoying life more than food

Before my weight loss surgery in June 2001, I weighed 397 pounds and wore a size 52/54. Since then, I've lost 223 pounds and wear a size 14/16. Before surgery, I had to take 12 different pills a day, treating everything from high blood pressure to high cholesterol (my total cholesterol was in the 600s), from diabetes to allergies, from ulcers to arthritis. Now, I take only one medication.

Looking back on my surgery, I wasn't prepared for the first several months to be so hard! The emotional aspect was explained to me by my surgeon, the people at the bariatric center, and others who had the surgery — and even though I listened, it just wasn't very high on my list of things to focus on. Questions like, "How long before I'm off my medications?" or "How long before I get below 200 pounds?" or "What about the extra skin?" were what I was thinking about. I was completely focused on things that were physical or visual — not emotional.

Knowing what I know now, I wish I'd spent more time before the surgery attending support-group meetings or reviewing personal stories online — helping myself understand the emotional part of this journey. If I hadn't had such wonderful support from my sister and

other family and friends, this experience would have been even harder. After all, when I had weight loss surgery, I lost my best friend — food — something that had been there for me since childhood and had been very, very loyal and consistent.

After the surgery, I kept reminding myself of a couple things I learned in the pre-op meetings:

✔ The surgery is a tool, not a miracle — use the tool to help yourself be disciplined.

✔ You'll find other things after your weight loss that you *will* enjoy as much as you enjoyed food.

The first one I didn't have trouble with — I did need help with discipline, and the surgery was the tool I needed. But the second one was a little hard for me to wrap my arms around. Enjoy something as much as I enjoy food? But guess what? It was true. There are several things that I enjoy now as much as I enjoy food.

I've known several people who've had the surgery since I had mine. Each time I wish I could take their hands and travel in time forward one or two years so they can see what they'll look and feel like. When you're 100 to 200 pounds

(continued)

overweight, that image of yourself feeling and looking good is almost impossible to see. Even remembering or knowing what that kind of happiness feels like is difficult. I try to tell people who are going through weight loss surgery that they'll still have emotional times — but the ratio of bad times to good times will flip-flop. Soon, the majority is good instead of bad!

And now, there's not a bad day that can't be brightened by shopping for a size 14 pair of jeans! When you've never worn a pair of jeans

in your life, and you've gone from a size 52/54 to a size 14/16, having an event such as shopping be a good thing is monumental. Finding those trade-offs is important. It's also important to be realistic and realize that the surgery can't remove all those years of bad habits. My surgeon just gave me a helpful tool so that I could see the end in sight and have the motivation to stay on track after the tool had done its part.

Cindy Phipps
Indianapolis, Indiana

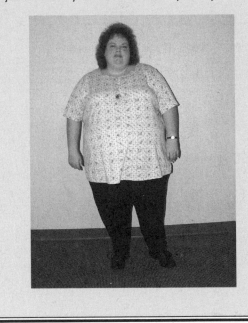 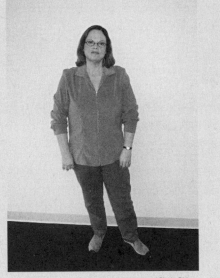

Photographs courtesy of Cindy Phipps

Chapter 15

Food for Thought: An Eating Plan for the Rest of Your Life

*I*n the first weeks and months after your surgery, you're focused on recovering and following your surgeon's guidelines and overcoming the hurdles and challenges along the way. After a while, though, you settle into a routine. The weight is coming off, and you eventually reach a healthy weight you can be happy with.

Your relationship with food and the importance of nutrition doesn't end at this point, however. Instead, nutrition is something you'll need to make a high priority for the rest of your life. This doesn't have to be a chore — in fact, when you see how good you feel when you give your body all the nutrients it needs, you'll want to continue doing exactly that.

In this chapter, we give you the information you need about protein, carbs, and fat; fill you in on the importance of water; let you know about the vitamins you'll need and the supplements to take; and give you some tips on incorporating this information into your daily life. We also leave you with fantastic, healthy recipes that we're sure will become favorites in the months and years to come.

The Building Blocks of Nutrition: Proteins, Carbs, and Fats

Just after your surgery, you'll be eating so little that you may think you're going to starve to death. For bypass, sleeve, and duodenal-switch patients, in the first few months, you'll probably eat between 400 and 800 calories per day. But as your hunger increases, so does the number of calories you eat. From about month 4 to month 12, you'll probably have about 1,000 to 1,200 calories per day. With gastric banding, you'll be eating less with every adjustment.

Try not to eat more than 1,200 calories per day until you're at your goal weight. Then increase your calories gradually until your weight is stable.

These calorie guidelines are generalizations and may need to be modified based on your height, the amount of exercise you do, and the recommendations of your own surgeon or dietitian.

Although calories are important, equally important is where you're getting those calories. The three building blocks of nutrition are protein, carbohydrates, and fats. In the following sections, we cover all three, letting you know how much of each you should strive for, and telling you which foods are the best sources of each (and which foods to avoid).

Ask your doctor or dietitian to check your resting energy expenditure (REE). This test measures how many calories you burn at rest per day and can help you guide your caloric intake for the day.

Protein: The whey to go

Protein is a major part of your diet after weight loss surgery. There are many ways to get your protein — and as many opinions on what the best source of protein is. We go into the details in this section, but the bottom line to keep in mind is that if you don't get enough protein, you'll lose muscle, your skin will appear saggy, and you'll show signs of aging.

When you eat protein, the protein is broken down into amino acids, which aid in the repair and building of muscles and the production of all the body's enzymes, including digestive enzymes. Amino acids are a part of good nutrition. Amino acids also are important for maintaining muscle mass and building muscles. You want to increase your muscle mass because muscles burn more calories than fat.

Looking at different sources of protein

When most people hear the word *protein,* they think of beef, chicken, fish, and eggs. Although these probably will be your main sources of protein, you can find protein in other places as well. Here's a list of some other great sources of protein you may want to try:

✔ **Soy products:** The most common examples of products that have soy protein are tofu and soy milk, both of which come from soybeans. Tofu is soybean curd; it comes in a variety of textures and consistencies, from the softest (which is silken) to extra firm. On its own, tofu has very little taste, but it will take the taste of whatever sauce it's cooked with.

Isolated soy protein is another great source of protein. It's formed by taking the fat and carbohydrates out of soybeans. What's left is a flavor-less, flourlike substance that consists of 90 percent to 95 percent pure protein. You can mix isolated soy protein with water, milk, or juice for a protein drink, or use it in cooking.

✔ **Whey protein:** When milk is turned to cheese, whey protein is separated out. Whey protein can be absorbed easily by the body, making it a very good source of protein. Whey protein is readily available as a protein powder in grocery stores, online, and in health-food stores.

Immediately following surgery, you may experience lactose intolerance and have trouble consuming whey-protein products. This normally goes away after a few months.

✔ **Meat substitutes:** If you're looking to cut down on your consumption of meat products because you're concerned about your cholesterol or because you're a vegetarian, meat substitutes can be your answer. Meat substitutes normally are found in the frozen-food section of most grocery stores. One form is known as textured vegetable protein (TVP). TVP resembles ground meat or chunks of meat (like stew meat). You can use it in recipes that call for these cuts of meat, substituting them in whole or in part. For example, you can make chili with half ground meat and half TVP.

Getting enough protein

How much is enough? Most surgeons and dietitians agree that the minimum daily requirement is 60 grams of protein. But in the first few months, you may struggle to consume that much. Protein supplements and bars can help. Some studies show that increasing your protein intake can maximize weight loss. Eating between 0.64 and 0.77 grams of protein per pound of body weight has shown the most benefit.

Table 15-1 provides some common protein sources and the amount of protein they provide, just to give you an idea of how much you'll need to consume to get up to the 60-gram mark.

Table 15-1	Protein Sources
Food	*Amount of Protein*
Egg, medium	6 grams
Milk, 8 ounces	6.3 grams
Fish, 3.5 ounces	21 grams
Cheddar cheese, 3.5 ounces	25 grams
Roast beef, 3.5 ounces	28 grams
Chicken, 3.5 ounces	25 grams
Deli meat, 3.5 ounces	13 grams
Tofu, 3 ounces	9 grams

Many weight loss surgery patients have problems eating protein; they complain that various meats feel like they get stuck going down. Here are some tips on what to buy and how to cook it to try to avoid these problems:

- **Buy the most expensive cuts of beef you can afford.** The more expensive the cut of beef, the more tender it is. And the more tender it is, the easier it will break down as you chew it. *Exception:* Buy the least expensive (chuck) ground beef, because it has a higher fat content, which makes the ground beef more tender and moist.

- **Cook beef to 140°F (60°C) and ground beef to 160°F (71°C).** Insert a meat thermometer (available at any cooking-supply store and some grocery stores) into the center of the meat to measure how warm it is.

- **Cook chicken only to a temperature of 165°F (74°C) for white meat and 185°F (85°C) for dark meat.** *Salmonella* — a nasty bacteria — is destroyed at 165°F (74°C), so you want to make sure to cook it to that temperature.

- **Cook pork only to a temperature of 150°F (66°C).** *Trichinosis* — another nasty bacteria, this one found in pork — is destroyed at 137°F (58°C).

- **Cook fish to a temperature of 140°F (60°C).**

- **Add moisture to your meat in whatever way you can, whether with broth or sauces.**

You may want to meet your daily protein requirements by drinking protein shakes or eating protein bars. Some of these shakes and bars are very high in protein and will satisfy your daily requirement in one or two servings. Just be aware of the number of calories and grams of sugar in shakes and bars — these all count toward your goal of maintaining your weight. Some protein powders that are high in protein and low in carbohydrates are

- ✔ Nectar
- ✔ Muscle Milk Lite (Sugar Free)
- ✔ Unjury
- ✔ Bariatric Advantage High Protein Meal Replacement
- ✔ Isopure

Protein bars meeting those requirements are

- ✔ Protein Fusion Bars
- ✔ Detour Bars
- ✔ PowerBar ProteinPlus Carb Select
- ✔ Revival Soy

A protein bar with more than 15 grams of sugar is really just a glorified candy bar.

Although protein shakes and bars may be a convenient way of consuming protein, they may not give you a feeling of fullness the way eating regular food will.

Several websites carry a great variety of protein shakes and bars, including www.bariatricadvantage.com and www.bariatriceating.com.

Carbs: Not all carbs are created equal

A *net carb* is a carbohydrate that is *metabolized* (used by your body) in a way that has an effect on blood sugar levels and the release of insulin. So, what does this mean exactly?

Protein not only helps you to heal and build muscle mass, but also acts as a natural appetite suppressant. Carbohydrates, on the other hand, actually increase your appetite. This is because, as you eat carbohydrates, the digestive process raises your insulin level. When the level of your blood sugar drops after your body has used the sugar, you have a tendency to crave more sugar to raise your blood sugar level again. The result is that your appetite will be stimulated by these carbohydrates.

Some carbohydrates don't raise your blood sugar level as high or as quickly as other types of carbohydrates. These are the carbohydrates that come from dietary fiber, glycerin, and sugar alcohol. Sugar alcohol comes from fruit and has half the calories of regular sugar. It's absorbed very slowly, which is why it doesn't cause your blood sugar level to spike. These carbs have no effect on your appetite and are actually better for you.

Although net carbs sometimes appear on the Nutrition Facts label, they don't always. So, you need to know how to calculate them for yourself. Here's how to calculate the number of net carbs in one serving of the food you're about to eat:

1. **Find the total number of carbohydrates listed on the Nutrition Facts label.**

2. **Subtract the number of grams of fiber, glycerin, and any grams of sugar alcohol (Maltitol or Lactitol).**

   The number that remains is referred to as the *net carbs* (sometimes referred to as *impact carbs,* because they have some impact on your blood sugar level). The net carbs are what you should count when determining how many carbs you've had each day.

To be very strict, you'll want to limit your net carbs to 20 to 30 grams per day. But remember: That determination should be made in consultation with a dietitian or your surgeon. Always follow your surgeon's and dietitian's recommendation over anything you read in this or any other book.

Even though you've had weight loss surgery, you still need to have five servings of fruits and vegetables daily — and fruits and vegetables are carbohydrates. Eating fruits and vegetables will provide you with fiber to aid in proper digestion, as well as important nutrients for good health.

Choose your fruits and vegetables carefully. For example, instead of having a serving of pineapple (which is high in calories and sugar), have a serving of strawberries. Initially, be wary of citrus fruits; their acidity may upset your stomach.

Eat whole fruits instead of drinking fruit juice — whole fruits have more fiber. If you want to drink fruit juice, dilute it nine parts water to one part juice so that you'll be drinking fewer calories and won't have to worry about the sweetness of the juice causing you to become nauseated.

Eating raw vegetables is much better than eating cooked ones, because the nutrients haven't been cooked away. Just be sure to chew them very carefully. You don't want anything to get stuck.

Fats: Good and bad

Fats are found in many of the foods you eat and are necessary to fuel your body. They add to the texture of food and make eating pleasurable. They're digested slowly and help to make you feel full longer. But not all fats are created equal. Some actually are good for you, and some are bad. Here are the main types of fats:

✔ **Saturated fats:** Saturated fats are solid at room temperature but become liquid when heated. They come from animal sources such as beef, butter, or cheese. They're known as the "bad" form of fat because they increase your cholesterol and triglyceride levels.

✔ **Polyunsaturated fats:** These fats are liquid at room temperature. They come from plants; you'll see them in safflower, sunflower, and corn oils. They're a healthier form of fat, because they help to lower cholesterol and triglyceride levels.

✔ **Monounsaturated fats:** Monounsaturated fats are the healthiest of the fats, because they help to lower your LDL ("bad") cholesterol. These fats come from olive and canola oils, peanuts, and avocados.

✔ **Hydrogenated fats:** Hydrogenated fats start out being healthy but because of processing end up being bad. These fats are processed so they'll last longer and not turn rancid. They're found in many packaged foods such as cookies, crackers, and margarines. Whenever you see something that's "partially hydrogenated" on the ingredient list, you know you're getting a hydrogenated fat (also referred to as a *trans fat,* which have been banned from use in certain states).

The American Heart Association recommends that you limit your fat intake to no more than 30 percent of the calories you eat. Therefore, if you eat a 1,200-calorie diet, no more than 360 calories should come from fat. One gram of fat equals about 9 calories, which means you shouldn't be eating any more than 40 grams of fat per day on a 1,200-calorie diet. If you have heart problems, your percentage of daily fat should be lower — 20 percent (about 27 grams of fat in a 1,200-calorie diet) or even 10 percent (13 grams of fat in a 1,200-calorie diet).

Supplementing Your Diet with Vitamins and Minerals

After you've had weight loss surgery, you'll need to commit to a regimen of vitamin and mineral supplements for the rest of your life. You'll be eating less food, and your body will be getting fewer nutrients — and, if you've had gastric bypass or duodenal switch surgery, you won't be absorbing as many nutrients because the food bypasses a part of your small intestine, where vitamins and minerals from food are absorbed.

So, you'll need to get these vitamins and minerals in the form of supplements. Otherwise, you'll end up with nutritional deficiencies — and you definitely don't want that.

How do you know if you're deficient in certain vitamins and minerals? Nutritional deficiencies don't show up immediately, so your doctor will need to check your blood levels a couple times within the first year after your surgery and then annually or semiannually thereafter, just to be sure you're getting everything you need.

The good news is that if you take your supplements and have your blood levels monitored by your surgeon, you can expect to stay healthy for the rest of your life. But being monitored by your surgeon is important — she'll know what to look for and what deficiencies look like.

Neither the Food and Drug Administration (FDA) nor any other government agency regulates vitamins and minerals, so buyer beware! For more information on vitamins, refer to *Vitamins For Dummies* by Christopher Hobbs, L.Ac., and Elson Haas, M.D. (Wiley).

The different forms of vitamins and minerals

Following surgery, you'll find yourself being very cautious about what you swallow, so the form in which you take your supplements will be very important to you. Here are the various forms that vitamins and minerals come in:

- ✔ **Pills:** When most people think of taking vitamins, they think of pills. You may start out using a chewable pill — maybe even a children's chewable vitamin — but as you become more confident, you'll need to graduate into adult supplements. Some vitamin pills are very large and will be very difficult for you to break down internally. Many adult vitamins and calcium supplements are in a chewable form; chewable fish oil supplements also are available. The best way to tell if you're absorbing vitamin pills is to have your blood levels checked and to evaluate how you're feeling.

- ✔ **Powders and liquids:** Several liquid vitamins are available — some are liquid when you buy them, and others are powdered and are mixed with water to become a liquid that you drink. The advantage of liquid vitamins is that they're more easily absorbed by your body than pills are. Liquid vitamins vary greatly in their taste — some taste quite good, and others are rather nasty, so shop around until you find one that tastes good to you.

- ✔ ***Sublingual* (under-the-tongue) vitamins:** Vitamins taken under the tongue are absorbed directly into your system and bypass your digestive system. B12 vitamins are readily available in a sublingual form.

- ✔ **Injection:** Vitamin B12 is sometimes given as a monthly injection. In cases of more serious anemia, iron injections may be called for.

Knowing which vitamins and minerals you'll need

As always, your surgeon and dietitian should be your first sources of information on which vitamins you should take. But in the following sections, we provide an overview of some of the vitamins you'll probably take, along with some info on why they're important.

Multivitamins

Take a good multivitamin so you'll get a variety of vitamins you'll be missing because you're eating (and possibly absorbing) less.

The labels on multivitamin bottles list the percentage of Recommended Dietary Allowances (RDAs). These are the minimum amounts of vitamins and nutrients needed for people who are in very good health. Be sure that the multivitamin you take has double the RDAs (or 200 percent) for each vitamin and mineral. Table 15-2 lists the RDAs to look out for.

Table 15-2	Recommended Dietary Allowances of Vitamins and Minerals
Vitamin	**RDA**
Vitamin A	10,000 IU
Beta-carotene	15,000 IU
Vitamin B1 (thiamine)	50 mg
Vitamin B2 (riboflavin)	50 mg
Vitamin B3 (niacin)	100 mg
Niacinamide	100 mg
Vitamin B5 (pantothenic acid)	100 mg
Vitamin B6 (pyridoxine)	50 mg
Vitamin B12	300 mcg
Biotin	300 mcg
Choline	100 mg
Folic acid	800 mcg
Inositol	100 mg
Para-aminobenzoic acid (PABA)	50 mg
Vitamin C with mineral ascorbates	3,000 mg
Bioflavonoids (mixed)	500 mg

(continued)

Table 15-2 *(continued)*

Vitamin	*RDA*
Hesperidin	100 mg
Rutin	25 mg
Vitamin D	400 IU
Vitamin E	600 IU
Vitamin K[1]	100 mcg
Essential fatty acids (EFAS)[2]	As directed on label
Minerals	RDAs
Calcium	1,500 mg
Chromium (GTF)	150 mcg
Copper	3 mg
Iodine[3]	225 mcg
Iron	18 mg
Magnesium	750 to 1,000 mg
Manganese	10 mg
Molybdenum	30 mcg
Potassium	99 mg
Selenium	200 mcg
Zinc	50 mg
Optional Supplements	Daily Dosages
Coenzyme Q10	30 mg
Garlic	As directed on label
L-Carnitine	500mg
L-Cysteine	50 mg
L-Lysine	50 mg
L-Methionine	50 mg
L-Tyrosine	500 mg
Lecithin	200 to 500 mg
Pectin	50 mg
RNA-DNA	100 mg
Silicon	As directed on label
Superoxide dismutase (SOD)	As directed on label

[1] *Use natural sources such as alfalfa and green leafy vegetables.*
[2] *Primrose oil, flaxseed oil, salmon oil, and fish oil are good sources.*
[3] *Kelp is a good source.*

Folic acid: It does a heart good

When you're shopping for a multivitamin, look for folic acid. A folic acid deficiency has been linked to heart disease and a greater risk of cancer. That said, you don't want to take more than 1,000 micrograms (mcg) of folic acid daily, because it may trigger vitamin B12 deficiency.

Here are some excellent natural sources of folic acid:

- Fruits
- Beef liver
- Dark green vegetables such as spinach, broccoli, and asparagus
- Peas
- Dried beans
- Cereal grains and breakfast cereals (which are fortified with folic acid)

Iron

Iron deficiency is the most common deficiency among weight loss surgery patients, although you don't need to take an iron supplement unless you're found to be deficient. Iron is important in making new red blood cells, improving brain function, improving immunity, and creating white blood cells. If you're not getting enough iron, you'll feel very tired.

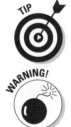

When you take an iron supplement, take vitamin C at the same time. It helps with the absorption of iron.

Don't take calcium and iron at the same time. The iron restricts the absorption of the calcium, so you should take them at least four hours apart.

Here are some natural sources of iron you can include in your diet:

- Blackstrap molasses
- Clams
- Dark green leafy vegetables
- Dried fruits
- Enriched and/or whole-grain breads and cereals
- Legumes
- Meat
- Nuts and seeds
- Oysters

- Pumpkin seeds
- Soybeans
- Tofu

Vitamin B12

We bet before weight loss surgery, you never thought to yourself, "Gee, I wonder if I'm getting enough B12." After weight loss surgery, getting enough B12 is a concern — vitamin B12 is the second most common deficiency (after iron) following weight loss surgery.

The *duodenum,* or the first part of the small intestine, is where the majority of vitamin B12 is absorbed. Because that part of the intestines is bypassed in gastric bypass and duodenal switch surgery, if you've had those types of surgery, you'll need to take a B12 supplement soon after surgery. Another reason that B12 is not well absorbed after weight loss surgery is because vitamin B12 needs a substance produced in the stomach called *intrinsic factor;* with the majority of the stomach bypassed or removed as in sleeve gastrectomy, intrinsic factor is less available, and the body doesn't absorb the B12 it needs.

So, why does vitamin B12 matter? B12 is important for proper nerve function, metabolism, and the production of red blood cells. Severe vitamin B12 deficiency can result in nerve damage. This deficiency takes years to show up, so your doctor should check your B12 levels for the rest of your life.

When shopping for vitamin B12, look for a liquid or sublingual form or take a monthly injection. The amount of supplement you'll need will depend upon your blood levels. But start with at least 500 mcg and then see after a few months how your body responds. (***Remember:*** Talk with your surgeon and dietitian and take their advice over anyone else's.)

Good food sources of vitamin B12 include the following:

- Eggs
- Fish such as tuna
- Fortified cereals, soy milk, and tofu
- Meat and meat products
- Poultry
- Shellfish
- Yogurt

Calcium

Calcium is important for the preservation of bone mass, regulating your heart rate, and blood clotting. It is essential for normal bone and tooth formation, overall growth, blood clotting, regulation of heart rate, and proper nerve transmission.

Here are some good sources of calcium found in foods:

- Almonds
- Broccoli
- Clams
- Cocoa
- Cottage cheese
- Dried fruit
- Legumes
- Milk
- Mustard greens
- Oysters
- Salmon
- Sardines
- Tofu
- Turnip greens
- Yogurt

Taking a daily calcium supplement is essential. People who are 19 to 50 years of age need 1,000 mg of calcium per day. Those older than 50 require 1,500 mg per day. Getting the required amount of calcium daily in the small amounts of food you're eating can be difficult. Therefore, supplements are a must.

There are several forms of calcium you can take (and scientists disagree on which is the best). Here are the two most common forms of calcium:

- **Calcium carbonate:** This is the form of calcium that is very often available as a calcium supplement. It is the least expensive and has the highest form of *elemental calcium* (the part of calcium that is usable and is available to be absorbed). Calcium carbonate requires an acidic environment to be absorbed. Normally, the gastric acid in the stomach provides this environment. With the reduced gastric acid in your small pouch following gastric bypass surgery and maybe also with a sleeve gastrectomy, you may not have enough acid in your stomach for calcium carbonate to be absorbed.

> ✔ **Calcium citrate:** Many agree that this is a more reliable form of calcium to take because it has no requirement for absorption. The elemental calcium in calcium citrate is lower than in calcium carbonate, but calcium citrate does not require an acidic environment in order to be absorbed.

Be sure that whatever calcium you take includes magnesium in a two-to-one ratio. In other words, there should be two parts calcium to one part magnesium. Vitamins C and D should be included as well; these aid in absorption.

Don't take iron at the same time you take calcium. The iron will interfere with your body's absorption of calcium. Separate when you take them by four hours.

Hydropower: The Role of Water

You may have rarely drunk water prior to surgery. So, now you may be thinking, "I got along well before without drinking water — I'll be fine after surgery." Unfortunately, that's not true. After surgery, you don't have the same capacity to eat, so you won't be getting the same amount of water from food, which is why you're so prone to dehydration after weight loss surgery.

How much

You'll have to get used to drinking water on its own. At a minimum, you should drink 64 ounces of water per day. You may need to drink even more water if you're physically active or weigh more. For a calculator of the amount of water you should drink, go to www.bottledwater.org/public/html/input1.html and click on the hydration calculator. When in doubt, consult your surgeon and/or dietitian.

Calcium banking

The calcium in your body that keeps your bones thick and strong is like a savings account. The calcium you get from food and calcium supplements is like a checking account. Your body requires calcium throughout the course of a day, and it takes the calcium from your supplements and food. When you aren't getting in enough calcium, your body pulls calcium from your bones and withdraws the calcium it needs. Your body does this automatically, and you have no idea how much calcium is being withdrawn from your bones. The more calcium that is withdrawn, the more susceptible you are to osteoporosis.

You don't have to limit yourself to water. You also can try drinks such as Gatorade, which has 50 calories per 8 ounces, or Crystal Light, which has 0 calories per 8 ounces. Try to shoot for calorie-free drinks whenever possible. If you're looking for a drink that has electrolytes like Gatorade (for example, if you're exercising and sweating a lot), but you don't want all the calories, try Propel; it has only 10 calories per 8 ounces. You can kill two birds with one stone: Isopure makes a drink that has 40 grams of protein per 20 ounces.

Why

Water serves so many functions that you can't live more than a few days without it. Water flushes toxins from your liver and kidneys. It regulates your body temperature and reduces the risk of many cancers by as much as 50 percent. It helps with your digestion and lubricates your joints. It allows you to store glycogen in your muscles, which provides you with energy.

Water takes up space in your pouch, so it will help eliminate hunger just by its volume. But water helps with hunger in another way: Whether you've had weight loss surgery or not, thirst is often confused with hunger. In other words, if you feel hungry, you may actually be thirsty instead.

When

After weight loss surgery, you have to drink water, but you can't have water when you eat. Be sure to wait 30 minutes before eating and 30 minutes after eating to have anything to drink.

Here's why you need to keep food and water separate:

- ✔ **If you drink before you eat, you'll fill up your new stomach with liquid and have no room for the food that you need to consume.** If you don't eat enough, you may find yourself hungry before you should be.

- ✔ **If you drink after eating, you'll wash the food out of your new stomach and you won't have a sustained feeling of being full.** You'll fill your new stomach with liquid, which empties faster than solid food, so in an hour, you'll feel hungry again. This gives you the urge to snack, which you want to avoid.

If you're feeling overwhelmed with keeping track of when you last ate and when you last drank, don't worry. Just do your best — keeping track of these things will eventually become second nature.

Which drinks to avoid

Caffeine is a diuretic, which means it makes you urinate. So, if you're trying to hydrate, drinking regular coffee or tea is not the best choice. Caffeine also can hurt your new stomach if you drink it in large amounts, so early on, cut back on caffeine or, if you can, eliminate it entirely.

Whether you call them soda or pop, carbonated beverages are hard to tolerate right after surgery, even if they're sugar-free. Here are a few reasons to avoid carbonated drinks:

✔ **Carbonation will give you more gas.** Even if you let a carbonated beverage sit until it's

flat, when you drink it, the heat of your body will release more carbonation, and the gas will come out one way or another. (You may have heard that your pouch will expand because of carbonation, but this is a theory that has never been proven.)

✔ **Some studies from the 1990s have suggested that the phosphoric acid found in sodas reduces the calcium in bones.**

✔ **Some studies indicate that some artificial sweeteners such as aspartame can make you hungrier.**

Bring a water bottle with you everywhere. Try to take a small sip every two minutes, all day long. You'll definitely get your fluid requirements in for the day if you do that. As time goes on, you'll drink more than the minimum, as you learn to eat and drink with your new stomach. *Remember:* Having weight loss surgery involves a lot of changes, and drinking enough water at the appropriate times is just one of them.

What's for Dinner? Eating Strategies for the Long Haul

Learning to control what you eat is the difference between success and failure after weight loss surgery. The first year may start out challenging, with nausea and difficulty getting food down. But eventually you get the hang of it. In fact, you may get the hang of it so much that you're finding that food is going down *too* well.

You may have a tendency to push the envelope. You're going month after month, and the pounds are falling off. You may wonder how much you can eat and still lose weight. You may want to just try eating more to see how much you can actually get away with. How many calories will it take until you stop losing weight? So, you get gutsy and eat more.

You may run into plateaus or just become complacent. This can be the beginning of the end of your weight loss. Here are some eating strategies to follow so you can reach your goal weight:

- ✔ **Remember that variety is key.** Don't eat the same foods every day. Variety can help keep you on your diet.

- ✔ **Use a food diary.** A food diary is a useful tool not only when you're losing weight but also when you're trying to maintain your weight. A diary helps keep you aware of what you're eating and whether you're tending toward grazing. Also, try to write down how you feel when you eat. That helps to track when you stray toward unhealthy eating behaviors.

- ✔ **Eat a healthy diet.** You have a small pouch and may think that, because you're eating so little, it doesn't matter what you eat. But it *does* matter. You may have a diet that consists of 1,000 healthy calories or a diet that consists of 1,000 unhealthy calories. You are what you eat. And although you may not be gaining weight, what you eat will determine such things as the energy you have and how free of fats your arteries are.

- ✔ **Understand that plateaus are a normal part of life.** Weight loss is not a straight line. You lose weight and then either stop or gain a little. The plateaus can be as long as three weeks in length. Be patient.

- ✔ **Plan your meals.** If you don't plan, you'll be tempted to *graze* (eat without planning to). People are generally prone to graze at the same time every day. Try to identify your weak times. If you're aware of when you're prone to grazing, you'll have an easier time resisting the urge.

- ✔ **Make sure you have enough fiber in your diet.** Fiber is not only healthy but filling.

- ✔ **Avoid fried food.** Grill, steam, or bake your foods instead.

- ✔ **Chew, chew, chew.**

- ✔ **Make every morsel you put in your mouth count.**

Regaining your appetite — without fear

After eating *simple carbohydrates* (such as sugar, white rice, or white bread), you may find that your blood sugar rises too quickly. This simple carbohydrate is broken down quickly into glucose, which causes a rapid rise in your blood sugar level as your body attempts to transport glucose. When your blood sugar level drops, you may experience cravings.

Cravings can be very scary. You probably believed that after you had surgery, you would never experience hunger again. Not so. Hunger is definitely a part of your life. The trick is managing it. Here are some tips for doing exactly that:

- ✔ **Stay away from simple carbohydrates.** These include foods like white breads, white rice, potatoes, pasta, and sweets.

- ✔ **If you're particularly sensitive, delay all carbohydrates to as late in the day as possible.**

- ✔ **Keep hydrated.** Remember that you may be mistaking hunger for thirst.

- ✔ **Don't get into the habit of grazing.** The best way to do this is to keep a food diary and become very conscious of what you're eating.

- ✔ **Be sure you're eating enough.** Some people are afraid to eat following their surgery — they're sure they'll regain their weight. But you need to be sure to eat a healthy diet and get the right amount of calories to maintain your weight.

Simple carbohydrates can cause late dumping or profound reactive hypoglycemia (meaning really low blood sugar) in gastric bypass patients long-term. You are hungry all the time because your blood sugar keeps falling from the carbs you are eating. Some of the other side-effects that patients with late dumping experience are sleepiness, forgetfulness, and feeling lightheaded to the point of passing out after eating carbs. These types of symptoms are called *neuroglycopenia* (meaning your brain gets low on sugar). Eating a diet high in protein with healthy carbs like vegetables and eating small meals often can help with this syndrome.

Following the rules your pouch sets

Keeping your new stomach small should be your lifelong objective. Your new stomach is vulnerable to stretching. If you've had gastric bypass surgery, you should also be concerned about stretching the *stoma* (the opening between the pouch and the small intestines).

Here are some tips to keep that pouch as small as possible:

- ✔ **Don't overeat.** Learn the signals that your body gives you to tell you you're full. You may feel a pain or pressure in the upper-chest area or you may feel as though you're about to throw up. Whatever the feeling is, be sure to heed it and stop eating. And in the future, try to stop eating *before* you feel that full.

- ✔ **Don't eat and drink at the same time.**

- ✔ **Don't eat foods that absorb a lot of water (such as rice).** After you eat these foods, they can continue to expand in your new stomach and stretch it.

Handling social situations

Many people's lives center around social situations — whether birthday parties, business lunches, or holidays. You may feel uncomfortable participating in these in the first months after your surgery, but eventually you'll be right back to normal, taking part in all the things you used to.

In the following sections, we help you maneuver two situations that cause weight loss surgery patients some anxiety: dining out and drinking alcohol.

Dining out

You may think that, after surgery, your restaurant days are over, but nothing is farther from the truth. Although you'll be very limited in the first few months, after that you'll find that you can do just fine in restaurants if you follow some of these tips:

- **Choose restaurants you know.** If you're familiar with the menu, you'll have some idea what the restaurant may have that you're able to eat.

- **Order an appetizer for your dinner.** Appetizers are often high in protein and easy to eat.

- **When in doubt, order soup or scrambled eggs.**

- **Though you may be tempted to order off the children's menu to get a smaller portion, avoid it because the choices aren't very healthy.** Spaghetti, pizza, or hot dogs are likely to be your typical options — and they're loaded with carbohydrates and fats.

- **If you see something on the menu that looks good, order it even though it's a full portion, and warn the waiter that you'll be eating very little and will need to take home most of your meal.** That stops the questions about what's wrong with your food.

- **Get used to doggy bags.** They'll be a regular part of your dining experience from now on.

Most restaurants have websites where you can look up their menus. Definitely do this. You don't want to arrive at the restaurant only to find that there's nothing for you to eat. Here are some notes on different kinds of restaurants to consider:

- **Buffets:** You may think your buffet days are over, but not so. You won't be able to load up your plate as you did before, but you still can enjoy buffet restaurants. The advantage is that you'll have control over every item on your plate, and you can see what you're getting. Most buffets offer a soup and a baked-fish choice. Just don't fall into the "big food" trap.

✔ **Fast food:** Guess what? Your fast-food days aren't over either. Many fast-food restaurants serve soups and chili. Eventually, you'll be able to have salads — just be wary of the dressing. There are more calories in dressings than in the sandwiches. Be sure to use the low-calorie selections.

✔ **Chinese:** Order carefully in Chinese restaurants. Many of the menu items have a lot of sugar in the sauces, which not only are full of calories but will cause you to dump (see Chapter 18). Most Chinese restaurants offer a white sauce, which is lower in calories, fat, and sugar. Always request that sauces be served on the side. Pass on all rice. It will expand in your pouch and is a simple carbohydrate. Also pass on the breaded and fried selections. Any of the other selections can be prepared steamed as opposed to sautéed — just ask your server.

✔ **Mexican:** Most Mexican dishes are very high in fat, but some selections are okay. Fajitas are a good choice if you eat the meat and vegetables and forgo the tortilla, sour cream, and guacamole.

✔ **Seafood:** Seafood restaurants offer excellent choices of baked and steamed seafood and fish.

✔ **Steak:** Many people have difficulty with steak following surgery. If you're able to eat steak, order the most tender cut of meat you can afford.

✔ **American:** In these restaurants, you'll find lots of variety. Be sure to speak up and say how you want things prepared. Ask the waitress how tender a cut of meat is and warn her that if it's tough, you'll have to send it back. Try out the fish selections and salads. If all else fails, request scrambled eggs.

✔ **Italian:** Italian restaurants serve great food other than pasta. Order the fish, chicken, or meatballs. Get a pasta fagioli! If you have to have pasta, go for the whole-wheat version and ask for an appetizer portion.

TIP

Getting carded

Some surgical practices provide their patients with a card to be used in restaurants. It explains that you've had surgery that limits your ability to eat a large amount of food, and it requests that you be permitted to order off the children's menu or to order half portions. It's up to the restaurant whether it will honor the card.

On one side of the card is normally the name and address of the practice and the surgeon, and on the other side is the request information. If your surgeon doesn't provide these cards, you can create your own restaurant card at `www.wlscenter.com/restaurant_card.htm`.

Handling alcohol

Each person has his or her own reasons for having weight loss surgery, but one of the more common reasons is so that you can live like "normal"-weighted people. And "normal"-weighted people sometimes drink alcohol. It's unrealistic to think that, after surgery, you'll never drink alcohol again. But you'll need to keep in mind some very specific guidelines when you do:

- ✔ **Alcohol dehydrates you, so be sure to drink extra water when you do drink alcohol, to make up for the dehydrating effects.**

- ✔ **Try to avoid your first alcoholic drink for as long as you can after your surgery.** Don't have a drink for at least the first six months. Alcohol provides you with empty calories, and you want your calories to count during that first year when you're concentrating so hard on losing every pound you can.

- ✔ **Have your first drink when you're at home in a safe environment.** You need to know how the alcohol will affect you before drinking in public. After weight loss surgery, one drink can be like having two or three!

- ✔ **Stay away from all sweet drinks.** They'll make you dump if you have had a gastric bypass (see Chapter 18). If you've had a different weight loss surgery procedure, drinking alcohol just gives you a bunch of empty calories (no nutrition and a bunch of sugar). Your daiquiri and margarita days are over.

- ✔ **Alcohol gets into your bloodstream much faster after surgery than it did before surgery, so the alcohol will hit you much harder.** Studies also have shown that it takes a little longer for your blood alcohol level to come down.

- ✔ **Never drink and drive.** The way that alcohol affects you after surgery will definitely impair your ability to drive.

Some patients after weight loss surgery become alcoholics. Perhaps it's because alcohol takes the place of food. Perhaps it's alcohol use as a different coping mechanism. Either way, it's critical to your overall health and weight maintenance that you assess how much alcohol you take in every day. If you have to drink every day, address why.

Although the American Heart Association says it's healthy for women to have one glass of red wine per day and for men to have two glasses of red wine per day, the effect of the wine is greater in weight loss patients. Be cautious with alcohol after the surgery and keep track of your drinking behavior. Make sure you're honest with your surgeon and dietitian about your alcohol intake.

Ten Healthy Recipes for the Rest of Your Life

You've finally reached the point in your journey when you're eating "normally" even though there were probably many times in the first few months when you didn't think you would ever enjoy eating again. These recipes are designed to show you that you can eat not only very healthy food but delicious food as well. The serving size is normally 4 ounces, but you may have leftovers in the beginning.

For more delicious and healthy recipes, check out *Weight Loss Surgery For Dummies Cookbook,* by Brian K. Davidson, David "Chef Dave" Fouts, and Karen Meyers, MS, RD/LD (Wiley).

Honey Chicken Stir Fry

Prep time: About 15 min • **Cook time:** 10 min • **Yield:** 6 servings (4 ounces each)

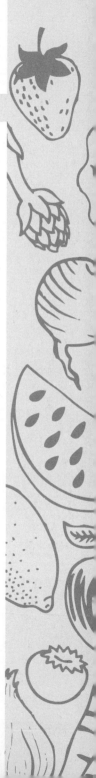

Ingredients	*Instructions*
4 teaspoons peanut oil	*1* In a large skillet, heat the oil over medium-high heat; add the chicken and sauté for 3 minutes.
1 pound boneless skinless chicken breast, cut ½-inch thick	
2 cups small broccoli florets	*2* Add the broccoli, onion, carrots, and mushrooms to the chicken and sauté for 5 minutes.
1 small onion, cut into thin strips	
1 medium carrot, cut into thin slices	*3* Add the honey, sesame oil, red pepper flakes, and soy sauce.
2 cups small mushrooms, cut in half	
¼ cup honey	*4* Stir until all the vegetables are glazed and the sauce is bubbly hot, about 1 minute.
1 teaspoon sesame oil	
¼ teaspoon crushed red pepper flakes	
2 tablespoons soy sauce	

Per serving: Calories 181 (From Fat 51); Fat 6g (Saturated 1g); Cholesterol 42mg; Sodium 358mg; Carbohydrate 16g (Dietary Fiber 2g); Protein 18g.

Tip: Make sure all the chicken is the same size so it will cook evenly.

Tip: This recipe is great served with brown rice and garnished with sesame seeds and chopped chives.

Vary It! You can use shrimp and scallops in this recipe if you prefer.

Floribbian Shrimp

Prep time: 30 min • **Cook time:** 10 min • **Yield:** 4 servings (4 ounces each)

Ingredients	Instructions
4 drops liquid smoke flavoring	**1** Combine in a medium mixing bowl the liquid smoke, honey, lime juice, and lemon pepper.
2 tablespoons honey	
1 tablespoon lime juice	**2** Add the shrimp and let it marinate for 30 minutes. After the shrimp has marinated, drain the shrimp and discard the marinade.
1 teaspoon lemon pepper	
1 pound medium shrimp, peeled and deveined	
2 teaspoons garlic, chopped	**3** In a 10-inch skillet over medium-high heat, add the garlic and olive oil.
1 tablespoon olive oil	
¼ cup heavy cream	**4** When the olive oil and garlic begin to sizzle, add the shrimp.
¼ teaspoon curry powder	
	5 Sauté for 4 to 5 minutes or until shrimp is pink in color.
	6 Add the heavy cream and curry powder and bring to a simmer. Let simmer for 3 minutes.
	7 Serve.

Per serving: Calories 178 (From Fat 89); Fat 10g (Saturated 4g); Cholesterol 188mg; Sodium 228mg; Carbohydrate 3g (Dietary Fiber 0g); Protein 18g.

Note: If you have to clean and devein your own shrimp, check out the figure in Chapter 10 for guidelines.

Tip: Always throw out your used marinades. Using a marinade more than once can cause extreme bacterial growth, which can contribute to food-borne illness.

Tip: Keep in mind that curry is a strong spice, and a little goes a long way. Garnish with a lime wedge and serve over whole-wheat pasta.

Vary It! This recipe is great with scallops.

Salmon Blush

Prep time: About 5 min • **Cook time:** 12 min • **Yield:** 4 servings (4 ounces each)

Ingredients	Instructions
1 tablespoon butter	*1* In a large sauté pan over medium-high heat, add the butter and olive oil.
2 tablespoons olive oil	
1 pound salmon fillets	*2* When the butter and oil are heated, add the salmon. Sauté for 5 to 8 minutes depending upon the thickness of the salmon, turning the salmon over every 2 minutes.
1 teaspoon garlic, chopped	
2 tablespoons capers	
¼ cup red wine	*3* Add the garlic, capers, wine, and cream. Bring to a simmer and let simmer for 4 minutes.
¼ cup heavy cream	
Salt and pepper, to taste	
1 tablespoon fresh parsley	*4* Add the salt, pepper, and parsley. Serve.

Per serving: Calories 343 (From Fat 229); Fat 26g (Saturated 8g); Cholesterol 110mg; Sodium 342mg; Carbohydrate 1g (Dietary Fiber 0g); Protein 26g.

Tip: Salmon when fresh has the scent of fresh-cut watermelon.

Tip: You can garnish with chopped red bell pepper and serve with a baked sweet potato. The sweetness from the baked sweet potato complements this dish nicely.

Vary It! For a change of pace, you can use other fish, such as grouper, sea bass, and mahi-mahi, in this recipe.

Spaghetti Veggies

Prep time: About 10 min • **Cook time:** 10 min • **Yield:** 4 servings (4 ounces each)

Ingredients	*Instructions*
3 tablespoons olive oil	*1* In a large sauté pan over medium-high heat, add the olive oil.
2 cloves garlic, minced	
1 small onion, chopped	*2* When the olive oil is heated, add the garlic and onion and sauté for 1 minute.
2 medium yellow squash, chopped	
2 medium zucchini, chopped	*3* Add the yellow squash, zucchini, and pea pods.
2 cups pea pods	
¼ cup lemon juice	*4* Sauté for 5 minutes.
Salt and pepper, to taste	*5* Add the lemon juice, salt, pepper, and basil and sauté for an additional 2 minutes.
½ bunch fresh basil, chopped	
½ pound whole-wheat spaghetti, cooked	*6* Toss in the cooked whole-wheat spaghetti and sauté for an additional 2 minutes. Serve.

Per serving: Calories 359 (From Fat 104); Fat 12g (Saturated 2g); Cholesterol 0mg; Sodium 157mg; Carbohydrate 58g (Dietary Fiber 13g); Protein 13g.

Tip: Garnish with fresh basil and serve with Pork Chardonnay (later in this chapter). Chicken, fish, or pork complement this side dish well.

Tip: Whole-wheat pasta is a better choice than pasta made from white flour, because whole-wheat pasta has more fiber.

Burgundy Pork

Prep time: About 5 min • **Cook time:** 6 min • **Yield:** 4 servings (4 ounces each)

Ingredients	Instructions
2 tablespoons olive oil	*1* In a large sauté pan over medium-high heat, add the olive oil.
Four 4-ounce pork loin chops, pounded ¼-inch thick	
1 teaspoon chili powder	*2* Season the pork medallions with chili powder, salt, and pepper.
1 teaspoon salt	
1 teaspoon fresh ground pepper	*3* When the olive oil is heated, add the seasoned pork medallions and sauté for 1 minute each side.
2 cloves fresh garlic	
2 tablespoons capers	*4* Add the garlic and capers and sauté for 2 minutes. Remove the pork.
½ cup burgundy wine	
	5 Deglaze the pan with the burgundy and reduce by half, about 2 minutes. Serve.

Per serving: Calories 227 (From Fat 121); Fat 13g (Saturated 3g); Cholesterol 67mg; Sodium 765mg; Carbohydrate 2g (Dietary Fiber 1g); Protein 24g.

Tip: Pork tenderloin is the most tender cut from a pig. Like beef tenderloin, this muscle is used the least, so it's especially tender.

Tip: Garnish with fresh parsley and serve with a fresh Caesar salad topped with fresh-cut strawberries.

Pork Chardonnay

Prep time: About 10 min • **Cook time:** 10 min • **Yield:** 4 servings (4 ounces each)

Ingredients	*Instructions*
½ **teaspoon salt**	*1* Salt and pepper the pork tenderloin cutlets.
½ **teaspoon pepper**	
Four 4-ounce pork loin chops, pounded ¼-inch thick	*2* Add the thyme and paprika to the flour and lightly coat the pork cutlets with the seasoned flour.
1 teaspoon dried thyme	
1 teaspoon paprika	*3* Place the olive oil in large sauté pan on medium-high heat.
2 tablespoons flour	
2 tablespoons olive oil	*4* When the olive oil is heated, add the coated pork cutlet and sauté for 2 minutes each side. Remove the cutlets and keep warm.
¼ **cup white wine**	
1 large tomato, chopped	*5* Add the white wine to deglaze the pan and reduce by half.
¼ **cup fresh mushrooms, sliced**	
¼ **cup scallions, chopped**	*6* Add the tomatoes, mushrooms, scallions, garlic, pork cutlets, and chicken stock to the pan.
½ **clove fresh garlic, chopped**	
¼ **cup chicken stock**	*7* Let the pork dish simmer for 5 minutes. The stock will thicken while cooking.

Per serving: Calories 245 (From Fat 124); Fat 14g (Saturated 3g); Cholesterol 55mg; Sodium 391mg; Carbohydrate 7g (Dietary Fiber 1g); Protein 23g.

Tip: Garnish with fresh diced tomatoes and serve over a bed of Spaghetti Veggies (see the recipe earlier in this chapter).

Tip: You can make this dish in advance and reheat it. This dish is great for family buffets. The sauce is light and keeps the pork moist and tender.

Chicken Dijon

Prep time: About 5 min • **Cook time:** 12 min • **Yield:** 4 servings (4 ounces each)

Ingredients	Instructions
1 pound boneless skinless chicken breast, pounded thin	**1** Season the chicken breast with the garlic powder, salt, and pepper.
1 teaspoon garlic powder	
1 teaspoon salt	**2** Heat the olive oil in a large sauté pan.
2 teaspoons cracked black pepper	**3** When the oil is hot, sauté the chicken on each side for 2 minutes.
1 tablespoon olive oil	
1 teaspoon basil	**4** Add the basil, thyme, and white wine.
1 tablespoon thyme	
¼ cup white wine	**5** Reduce the white wine by half.
¼ cup heavy cream	**6** Add the heavy cream and mustard. Bring to a light simmer, and simmer for 4 minutes. Serve.
1 tablespoon Dijon mustard	

Per serving: Calories 217 (From Fat 108); Fat 12g (Saturated 5g); Cholesterol 83mg; Sodium 738mg; Carbohydrate 3g (Dietary Fiber 1g); Protein 24g.

Tip: Garnish with a lemon wedge and fresh chopped parsley and serve with fresh steamed green beans.

Vary It! You also can use boneless skinless chicken thighs, as well as shrimp, scallops, or veal.

Surf-and-Turf Kabobs

Prep time: About 15 min • **Cook time:** 7 min • **Special equipment:** Eighteen 4-inch wooden skewers • **Yield:** 4 servings (6 pieces of beef and 12 pieces of shrimp per serving)

Ingredients	Instructions
48 medium shrimp, peeled and deveined	*1* In a large mixing bowl, combine all the ingredients and mix well.
1½ pounds beef tenderloin, cut into twenty-four 1-inch cubes	*2* Place 4 shrimp on each of 12 skewers and 4 beef cubes on each of 6 skewers.
2 teaspoons granulated garlic	
1 teaspoon salt	*3* Place the skewers over medium coals on a grill, and cook for 7 minutes or until the shrimp is fully cooked. Serve.
1 teaspoon black pepper	
1 teaspoon onion powder	
1 teaspoon chili powder	
1 teaspoon thyme	
2 tablespoons olive oil	

Per serving: Calories 407 (From Fat 182); Fat 20g (Saturated 6g); Cholesterol 216mg; Sodium 775mg; Carbohydrate 3g (Dietary Fiber 1g); Protein 51g.

Tip: You can easily make your own horseradish sauce by adding 2 tablespoons of horseradish and 1 teaspoon granulated garlic to 1 cup mayonnaise.

Vary It! You also can bake at 350°F (177°C) for 15 minutes or sauté over medium-high heat for 8 minutes.

Ricotta Chicken

Prep time: About 15 min • **Cook time:** 20 min • **Yield:** 4 servings (5 ounces each)

Ingredients	*Instructions*
½ cup ricotta cheese	*1* Preheat oven to 350°F (177°C).
3 tablespoons pine nuts	*2* In a large bowl, combine the ricotta cheese, pine nuts, basil, thyme, garlic, sun-dried tomatoes, and artichoke heart. Mix well.
2 tablespoons fresh basil, chopped	
1 tablespoon fresh thyme, chopped	*3* Lay the pounded chicken breast flat and divide the cheese mixture evenly.
1 teaspoon garlic, chopped	
2 tablespoons sun-dried tomatoes, chopped	*4* Spread the cheese mixture over the top of the chicken breast and roll the chicken breast tightly.
1 artichoke heart, chopped	*5* Place the chicken seam side down into a baking pan.
1 pound boneless skinless chicken breast, pounded ¼-inch thick, being careful not to tear the meat	*6* Pour the white wine into the baking pan with the chicken, and add the salt and pepper.
½ cup white wine	*7* Bake at 350°F (177°C) for 40 minutes or until done and juices run clear. Serve.
Salt and pepper, to taste	

Per serving: Calories 222 (From Fat 90); Fat 10g (Saturated 4g); Cholesterol 79mg; Sodium 283mg; Carbohydrate 4g (Dietary Fiber 1g); Protein 28g.

Tip: Garnish with sun-dried tomatoes and serve with spaghetti squash.

Tip: You can prepare this dish a day or two in advance and store it in the refrigerator until you're ready to bake and serve it.

Mandarin Orange Salad

Prep time: About 10 min • **Cook time:** 0 min • **Yield:** 8 servings (4 ounces each)

Ingredients	*Instructions*
4 cups romaine lettuce, chopped	Place all ingredients into a large bowl and mix well. Serve.
1 cup mandarin oranges	
½ cup pecans, chopped	
¼ cup scallions, chopped	
½ cup plum tomatoes, chopped	
½ small cucumber, peeled and chopped	
¼ cup fresh strawberries, pureed	
¼ cup raspberry vinegar	
3 tablespoons vegetable oil	
¼ cup Gorgonzola cheese, crumbled	

Per serving: Calories 253 (From Fat 205); Fat 23g (Saturated 3g); Cholesterol 6mg; Sodium 8mg; Carbohydrate 12g (Dietary Fiber 4g); Protein 4g.

Tip: Avoid iceberg lettuce — it has very little nutritional value. Better choices are Romaine lettuce, Boston lettuce, baby field greens, and fresh spinach. To ensure that the lettuce doesn't get soggy, don't toss the salad until you're ready to serve it.

Vary It! You can add protein (for example, shrimp or chicken) to top this delicious salad.

Chapter 16

Getting It in Gear: Making Exercise Part of Your Routine

In This Chapter

▶ Understanding the importance of exercise

▶ Deciding whether to exercise at a gym, with a trainer, or on your own

▶ Choosing an exercise that's right for you

▶ Staying motivated

L arger people face special challenges when trying to be active. You may not have exercised in a while or you may have exercised in the past with poor results. You may not be able to bend or move in the same way that other people can. You may feel self-conscious being physically active around others. You may have trouble finding clothes and equipment for exercising. Facing these challenges isn't easy, but you *can* conquer them!

In this chapter, we fill you in on the benefits of exercise — and there are many of them, in addition to helping with weight loss. We also give you the scoop on working out at gyms, with personal trainers, and on your own. Your first activity will be walking, but you'll also find some suggested activities that will meet your body's exercise needs — you can choose the ones that you like the most, or try out a few you've never done before. Finally, we help you stay motivated when the going gets tough.

In order to lose weight — whether you've had weight loss surgery or not — you need to burn more calories than you take in (from food and drinks). To burn 1 pound of fat, you need to burn 3,500 calories. So, if you want to lose 1 pound of fat in one week, you need to burn 500 more calories per day than you're taking in. Your surgery will help you with reducing your caloric intake, but you still need to get off the couch and get moving in order to achieve a lasting weight loss and stay healthy and strong.

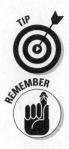

Through your surgeon's office, you may be able to get some help from exercise physiologists or certified personal trainers who have experience working with obese people, both before and after weight loss surgery. Ask your surgeon about these services.

Be sure to check with your doctor to find out when you're physically ready to start exercising. If you try to do too much too fast, you could do more harm than good.

What's in It for Me? Knowing the Benefits of Exercise

A regular and moderate exercise program can do the following:

✔ Speed up your recovery from surgery.

✔ Enhance your body's immune system.

✔ Help your body burn fat.

✔ Improve your self-esteem and confidence.

✔ Increase your strength.

✔ Boost your energy levels.

✔ Reduce your appetite and improve digestion.

✔ Help your heart and lungs work better.

✔ Decrease your stress and improve your mood.

✔ Build and preserve healthy muscles, bones, and joints.

✔ Prevent injury.

✔ Reduce depression and anxiety.

✔ Help control blood pressure and blood sugar.

✔ Improve flexibility.

✔ Improve sleep.

✔ Improve sexual satisfaction.

✔ Improve overall quality of life.

TECHNICAL STUFF

Metabolism: What it is and how to improve it

Basal metabolic rate (BMR) is a measure of the energy your body uses to maintain vital functions, such as breathing and blood circulation. BMR is what most people are referring to when they talk about metabolism. The higher your basal metabolic rate, the more calories you burn.

Metabolic rates vary from one person to another and are affected by many factors, such as sex, age, weight, height, muscle mass, and hormones. Metabolic rates are higher in tall, thin people; children; and pregnant women. Muscle mass actually increases the rate of your metabolism.

As people age, their body composition changes — they lose muscle mass. But regular physical activity can preserve lean body mass and may reverse the negative changes in body composition that are associated with age.

In addition to being affected by age, metabolism can be lowered by chronic dieting. Typically, when people diet, they lose lean muscle mass along with fat. Losing lean muscle mass lowers your metabolic rate. When dieting is over, and a more normal eating pattern returns, the metabolic rate remains lowered, and the person gains that weight back faster — but instead of gaining muscle mass, fat is what comes back. (Sound familiar?)

Luckily, this is not a hopeless scenario: You can increase your basic metabolic rate by increasing muscle mass, which you can do through weight training. Exercise burns calories while you're exercising, as well as increasing metabolism for several hours after exercise. Weight training can cause an increase in lean muscle tissue, which raises your resting metabolic rate.

A quick and easy way to estimate your metabolism is to multiply your current weight by 10 if you're a woman or 11 if you're a man — the number you get is the number of calories you burn in a given day without any activity.

Or, if you're up for doing a little math, try the following formulas:

> **Women:** $655 + (4.3 \times \text{weight in pounds}) + (4.7 \times \text{height in inches}) - (4.7 \times \text{age in years})$

> **Men:** $66 + (6.3 \times \text{weight in pounds}) + (12.9 \times \text{height in inches}) - (6.8 \times \text{age in years})$

For example, Mary is 40 years old, is 5'5" tall, and weighs 175 pounds. So $655 + (4.3 \times 175 \text{ pounds}) + (4.7 \times 65 \text{ inches}) - (4.7 \times 40 \text{ years}) = 1{,}525$ calories. The minimum number of calories Mary's body needs to function is 1,525. If she exerts herself in any way at all (even getting out of bed and walking around the house), her body will use more than 1,525 calories.

As you add muscle from strength training, your resting metabolism will increase, so you'll burn more calories all day. For each pound of muscle you gain, you'll burn 35 to 50 more calories daily. So, for example, if you gain 3 pounds of muscle and burn 40 extra calories for each pound, you'll burn 120 more calories per day, or approximately 3,600 more calories per month. That equates to a loss of 10 to 12 pounds in 1 year. *Remember:* Reducing calories in addition to exercising is the best way to lose weight.

As if all of that weren't enough, becoming physically active may help you live longer and reduce your risk of diabetes, heart disease, stroke, high blood pressure, osteoporosis, and colon and other cancers. If you have any of these health problems, being physically active may help to improve them.

After surgery, your body will be losing weight rapidly. As a result, it goes into a panic state and tries to hold on to stores of fat to prevent starvation. Instead of burning fat, your body will start to feed off of muscle tissue. Loss of muscle tissue will weaken the muscle and possibly put undo stress on other parts of your body. It also will adversely affect your metabolism (see the nearby sidebar). Regular exercise and a proper diet will combat these problems, helping your body burn fat instead of muscle.

Working Out at a Gym, with a Trainer, or On Your Own

When you're starting an exercise program, you can decide to work out at a gym or at home, with a personal trainer or on your own.

Your physician and members of your support group will be able to direct you to fitness professionals who can work with you before and after surgery. Many surgical practices even have exercise physiologists or certified personal trainers on staff; if yours doesn't, your surgeon can recommend people in your area.

Fitness professionals are a great resource for advice and guidance on proper exercise and health clubs that cater to larger people. They also can provide you with personal training services, or recommend equipment to buy if you're training at home.

You don't have to choose one or the other (home or gym, alone or with a trainer). If you want, you can start by working with a personal trainer in the privacy of your home. Then, when you're comfortable with the routine, you can keep it up on your own. And when you're ready to work out in a gym, you can make that transition. Or you could start in a gym and then transition toward working out at home. The best approach is the one that will keep you exercising regularly.

Gyms

A gym may or may not be for you, and all gyms are not the same. If you want to join a gym, shop around for one where you feel at ease. Make a list of the gyms in your area — being sure to focus on those that aren't so far away from your home or work that you'll use that distance as an excuse not to go — and then visit the gyms and ask the employees the following questions:

- ✔ Can the exercise machines or benches support larger people?

- ✔ Is the fitness staff experienced working with people of larger sizes?

- ✔ Do you offer a trial period so I can see how I like the facilities before I sign up?

- ✔ How much does it cost to join?

- ✔ What are the hours the gym is open?

- ✔ What fitness classes do you offer and are the classes included in the cost of membership?

- ✔ How busy does the gym get, and what times are the busiest?

Take a tour of the gym to see if you're comfortable in the environment and your surroundings.

Personal trainers

If you're new to exercise, beginning with professional instruction is a good idea. A personal trainer can build a routine for you that you can do at home or in the gym. You don't need to see a trainer for every exercise session. Four preliminary visits with a trainer may be enough to get you to a point where you can continue on your own. You also may consider periodic updates with the trainer.

If you're considering hiring a trainer, make sure he has worked with other people who've either gone through weight loss surgery or been severely obese and that he has delivered the results you're looking for. Finding an instructor who is willing not only to work with you, but also to educate you, is important. You'll also want an instructor who is friendly and promotes a fun environment for exercising.

Here are questions to ask trainers either in person or over the phone before hiring them:

- ✔ **Can you provide me with references?** Find out if the trainer has trained any weight loss surgery patients or people who were severely obese. A good trainer should be happy to provide you with names and numbers of clients you can contact.

- ✔ **How do you help your clients reach their goals?** The trainer's answer to this question will give you an idea of how she'll work with you and what her exercise and training philosophy is.

✔ **What organization(s) are you certified by?** Some reputable certification associations include the National Strength and Conditioning Association (NSCA; www.nsca-lift.org), the American College of Sports Medicine (ACSM; www.acsm.org), and the American Council on Exercise (ACE; www.acefitness.org). Many other associations certify personal trainers. Of course, certification — no matter what the organization — doesn't guarantee a quality instructor. Although certification is important, you'll want to use it in combination with the other information that you're collecting.

✔ **What is your fee and how do you expect payment?** Prices for personal fitness instruction vary widely based on where you live and the trainer's qualifications and experience. If the trainer is meeting you at your home, expect to pay slightly more than you'd pay if you meet at a gym.

Make sure you choose a trainer with whom you feel comfortable. You want someone whose personality is a good match with yours. And don't be afraid to switch trainers if the first one you choose doesn't end up working out.

Home

If you have trouble getting to a regular class, or if you just can't stand the thought of exercising in front of other people, home exercise is for you. You don't need benches or bars to start weight training at home. Some exercises require no equipment at all.

Make sure you know the correct posture and that your movements are slow and controlled. For a great primer on exercising, including tips on setting up a mini-gym in your own home, check out *Fitness For Dummies,* 4th Edition, by Suzanne Schlosberg and Liz Neporent (Wiley).

If you want to exercise at home and you're on a budget, here are some suggestions:

✔ Use objects from the pantry, such as soup cans, instead of buying hand-held weights.

✔ Consider buying secondhand equipment. You'll find weights and other equipment for sale in your local paper, in used sporting goods stores, and at online auction sites such as eBay (www.ebay.com).

✔ If you can't afford a class, buy an exercise DVD.

As you get into better shape, consider purchasing a few inexpensive pieces of equipment. Any sporting goods store should have a selection of dumbbells, or check out SPRI (www.spriproducts.com) for vinyl-coated dumbbells you can order online. Women should start with a pair of 2- or 3-pound weights; men, with 5- or 10-pound weights. Light weights that can be strapped to your feet or ankles are convenient as well. You also can look for adjustable dumbbells, to which you can add metal disks as your strength improves.

Before you buy a home gym, check its *weight rating* (the number of pounds it can support) to make sure it's safe for your size.

Looking At the Different Types of Exercise

When your initial recuperation from surgery is complete and your doctor says it's okay for you to exercise, it's important to pick exercises or activities you think you may enjoy. But no matter which ones you choose, you need to make sure that your exercise routine includes the two major forms of exercise: aerobic and anaerobic. Read on to find out why.

Knowing what to wear

Exercising is a lot more fun if you're wearing the right clothes. We're not talking fashion or style here — we're just talking clothes that were meant to be worn during exercise.

Start by wearing loose-fitting, comfortable clothing, made of fabrics that absorb and remove sweat from your skin.

If you're a woman, be sure to wear a good athletic bra — it'll give you more support than the one you wear for everyday, nonstrenuous activity.

Never wear rubber or plastic suits (once a major weight-loss fad); they hold the sweat on your skin and may cause your body to overheat.

Be sure to find a good pair of supportive athletic shoes for weight-bearing activities.

And top it all off by wearing sweatproof or waterproof sunscreen when your exercise takes you outdoors — whether in winter or summer, cloudy weather or sunshine.

Aerobic exercise

Aerobic exercise is exercise that gets your heart pumping. It helps your heart and lungs work better. As you increase your heart rate and your metabolism, your body will burn more fat.

When you're starting an aerobic exercise program, be sure to pace yourself. If you're exhausted, feel chest pains, or experience dizziness, stop and notify your doctor right away.

Build up gradually. Your body needs time to get used to your new activity. Any increase in your physical activity — no matter how small — can make a difference.

Knowing how hard to work

Your goal is to work within 60 percent to 75 percent of your maximum heart rate. Never go above 85 percent of your maximum. If you start approaching the upper limits, slow down and lower the intensity of your exercise.

So, how do you know what your maximum heart rate is? Subtract your age from 220. That's your maximum heart rate. Then, to determine the range you want to be working in, multiply times 0.6 for the low end of the range, and 0.75 for the high end of the range. For example, if you're 40 years old, you would calculate your target heart rate as follows: $220 - 40 = 180$ (your maximum heart rate). Multiply $180 \times 0.6 = 108$ (the minimum number of beats per minute you're targeting during aerobic exercise). Then multiply $180 \times 0.75 = 135$ (the maximum number of beats per minute you're targeting during aerobic exercise).

In order to find your heart rate, of course, you need to take your pulse. You can take your pulse for a full minute, or you can take it for 15 seconds and multiply that number times 4.

We recommend buying a heart-rate monitor to wear during your aerobic activity — using a heart-rate monitor is much easier than taking your pulse by hand and doing the math. You can find different models in sporting goods stores and online. A pedometer or a bodybugg (www.bodybugg.com) are excellent at keeping track of how many steps you take and how active you are. Some of the newer devices also can measure or convert your steps into the number of calories you burned.

Knowing how long to work

A good aerobic starting point is 12 minutes at a low to moderate intensity (60 percent to 75 percent of your maximum heart rate; see the preceding section), using a comfortable movement such as walking or pedaling a stationary bike. Be sure to warm up and cool down (see the following section) in addition to doing your aerobic activity; your entire workout session may last 16 or 17 minutes at first, including the warm-up and cool-down.

As you exercise more often, your heart becomes more efficient. Increase your aerobic activity slowly, just enough to present a new challenge. Your goal is to try to keep your heart rate in that 60 percent to 75 percent range for at least 20 consecutive minutes. Be sure to add additional time for warm-up and cool-down (which may bring your total time to at least 30 minutes). Do this at least three times per week.

Work your way up to 30 minutes of aerobic exercise (not counting the warm-up and cool-down) a few times per week. Then you can increase the challenge by varying the speed, intensity, incline, or workload depending upon the aerobic option you choose.

The current government guidelines regarding exercise call for 60 minutes of moderate to vigorous exercise most days to prevent weight gain and 60 to 90 minutes most days for weight loss.

Use the talk test to quickly determine if you're exercising too hard: If you're so breathless that you can't talk, ease up right away.

Warming up and cooling down

Warming up gets your body ready for action. Just as you need to prepare your car's engine for a trip, you need to prepare your heart the same way. The purpose is to slowly increase your heart rate to your personal training level, warm your muscles, and help prevent injuries. Spend a few minutes warming up for any physical activity.

You can do any of the following activities for a few minutes to warm up:

- ✔ Walking at a casual pace (If walking is your aerobic activity of choice, just walk slower for the first few minutes.)
- ✔ Marching in place
- ✔ Stationary bicycling
- ✔ Shrugging your shoulders
- ✔ Swinging your arms

For your cool-down, slow down little by little. If you've been walking fast, walk slowly or stretch for a few minutes to cool down. You also can repeat the warm-up and stretches you did before you exercised. Before you shrug it off and figure you don't need to cool down, keep in mind that cooling down may protect your heart, relax your muscles, and prevent injury.

Stretching

Stretching your muscles before and after every workout is important. It prepares your muscles for a workout and cools down your muscles after you're finished. Stretching will help you have a more effective workout and decrease your risk of injury. Stretching will also help you to

- Become more flexible
- Feel more relaxed
- Improve your blood flow
- Burn calories
- Keep your muscles from getting tight after doing other physical activities

You don't have to set aside a special time or place to stretch. At home or at work, stand up, push your arms toward the ceiling, and stretch. Stretch slowly and only enough to feel tightness, not pain. Hold the stretch, without bouncing, for about 30 seconds. Check out *Fitness For Dummies,* 4th Edition, by Suzanne Schlosberg and Liz Neporent (Wiley), for additional stretches.

Yoga

The word *yoga* comes from ancient Sanskrit and means "to join" or "to yoke," which relates to the philosophical belief in the joining of the mind, body, and spirit. By practicing yoga, you can deeply connect to your innermost self through a form of mindful exercise involving postures called *asanas,* controlled breathing called *pranayama,* and meditation.

Yoga is about feeling centered, emotionally and spiritually. The postures strengthen your body, the meditation sharpens your focus, and the breathing calms your mind and heals your body.

When the three are in harmony, the results are improved fitness, flexibility, stress management, relaxation skills, mental clearness, and overall well-being.

Classes usually are performed barefoot on a nonslip yoga mat in comfortable fitness wear. There are many different styles of yoga. If you're new to yoga, begin with hatha yoga, which is the basic form of the classic postures and the foundation for all the other styles of yoga.

You can find yoga DVDs, or you can take a class at your gym or health club.

Be sure to warm up a bit *before* you stretch — if you stretch cold muscles, you may injure yourself.

If you want to get even more stretching in, check to see whether your local fitness center offers yoga, ta'i chi, or other stretching classes. These classes help you breathe deeply, relax, and reduce stress. You may want to start with gentle classes, like those aimed at seniors.

Choosing an aerobic activity

You can choose from all different kinds of activities to get the aerobic workout you need. And if you like variety, you can try several different activities and rotate among them from day to day.

Here are some popular types of aerobic exercise:

- **Walking:** After surgery, you'll want to start with walking. When you first start walking, in the days immediately following your surgery, you'll be very tired and you won't be able to do much. But doing the walking your surgeon recommends is important — walking improves the healing process and helps prevent blood clots. You can use walking as a lifelong activity, increasing your speed as your fitness improves.

- **Aerobics:** You can do aerobics workouts in classes at a gym or using a DVD. Either way, they can be a great way to get your heart rate up.

- **Zumba:** A Latin dance-based fitness routine where you can dance your way to health. Sounds great! Zumba incorporates aerobic and resistance training. Many gyms teach classes, or you can buy DVDs for home use.

- **Pilates:** You can take classes or buy DVDs for this great method of building your core. Pilates is a system of exercises that help stabilize your core strength and your spine, and then works on resistance to increase your strength.

- **Core workouts:** There are many forms of core workouts; one example is Core Fusion. Many gyms have core-building classes. You can buy DVDs for this excellent method to improve your health and increase your BMR.

- **Swimming or water aerobics:** If your feet or joints hurt when you stand, non-weight-bearing activities such as swimming may be a great option for you. Swimming and water workouts place less stress on your joints because you don't have to lift or push your own body weight. If you don't know how to swim, no problem — you can perform shallow-water or deep-water exercises without swimming. Many swim centers or gyms offer classes in water workouts. Check with the pools and gyms in your area to find the best water workout for you.

✔ **Cardio kickboxing:** As with aerobics, you can take kickboxing classes at a gym, or you can find kickboxing DVDs.

✔ **Stair climbing or using a stair-climber machine:** Climbing stairs is a great way to raise your heart rate, and the incline or decline will stimulate your leg muscles from different angles.

✔ **Jogging:** When you're able to get your heart rate up by walking alone, and after the weight has come off, you may want to intersperse jogging with walking, and maybe even move entirely to jogging.

Keep in mind that jogging can be rough on your ankles and knees — you can start jogging a little after you've lost a substantial amount of weight (at least 50 pounds), as long as your joints can take it.

✔ **Training on an elliptical machine:** If you're exercising at a gym or health club and you have joint or back problems, an elliptical machine may be perfect for you. As with all machines, make sure you have a trained professional demonstrate the proper way to use the equipment if you haven't used it before.

✔ **Bicycling or stationary cycling:** You can bicycle indoors on a stationary bike or outdoors on a road bike. Biking doesn't stress any one part of the body — your weight is spread between your arms, back, and hips.

You may want to use a recumbent bike. On this type of bike, you sit low to the ground with your legs reaching forward to the pedals. This may feel better than sitting upright. The seat on a recumbent bike is also wider than the seat on an upright bike, which may feel better.

For biking outdoors, you may want to try a mountain bike. These bikes have wider tires and are heavy. You also can buy a larger seat to put on your bike. Make sure your bike has a weight rating at least as high as your own weight.

✔ **Spinning:** Spinning is a high-intensity group cycling workout led by an instructor who uses speed drills and visualization. Done in classes on special stationary bicycles, spinning doesn't put stress on the body and burns plenty of calories. Spinning bicycles have special weighted flywheels that make you feel like you're actually cycling. Beginners are in classes with experts, because each person controls the tension on his cycle; however, before taking a spinning class, you should be able to use a stationary bicycle for 30 minutes at moderate intensity.

✔ **Rowing:** Rowing can be done in the gym on a machine or in the water in a boat. This is an excellent way to get the blood pumping and work your upper-body muscles.

One of the easiest ways to exercise is to bring it into your daily life. You don't have to plan all your physical activities — you can make small changes to make your day more physically active and improve your health:

- ✔ Take the stairs instead of the elevator.

- ✔ Park at the far end of the parking lot.

- ✔ Hide the TV remote control and force yourself to get up to change the channel — or better yet, get off the couch and go for a walk.

- ✔ Get up and stretch and walk around your office as frequently as possible.

- ✔ Instead of sending an e-mail or making a phone call, walk to your co-worker's desk.

- ✔ Cruise around the shopping mall a number of times before starting to shop.

- ✔ Walk to your kids' school to pick them up instead of driving — they'll get the added bonus of walking home with you and getting some physical activity themselves.

- ✔ Stand up while talking on the phone.

- ✔ March in place during TV commercials.

If you can do only a couple of these activities, it's okay. Remember to appreciate what you can do, even if you think it's a small amount. Moving any part of your body, even for a short period of time, can make you healthier.

Doing chores like mowing the lawn, raking leaves, gardening, and cleaning the house also may improve your health. But in general, you'll want to use these chores to supplement your exercise regimen, not replace it.

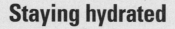

Staying hydrated

Drinking plenty of water keeps your body working properly, helps you stay energized, and allows you to work out longer. Try to drink 16 ounces of cool water two hours before exercise. Then drink as much as you can while you're exercising, shooting for at least another 16 ounces during your workout.

Sports drinks (like Gatorade or POWERade) are okay, but they can be high in calories and

sugar. Sports drinks do come in zero-calorie or low-calorie options, so check the labels. Cool water is still your best bet. Carry around a water bottle as you exercise and take a sip every few minutes.

Depending on how strenuous your daily routine is, you may need to drink as much as 96 ounces of water in a given day, but shoot for at least 64 ounces.

Anaerobic exercise

Anaerobic exercise — also known as strength training, weight training, or resistance training — builds strong muscles and bones. Anaerobic exercise is vital to maintain or even increase lean muscle mass. Getting stronger will enable you to better perform daily activities that require lifting, pushing, and pulling. Getting stronger also can help prepare you for other kinds of physical activity. You can train at home or at a fitness center.

You can start with a hand weight as light as 1 pound and increase the weight as you gain strength. When it comes to building strength, what matters most isn't so much the weight but performing the exercise correctly.

When your body adapts to that weight and that motion, you need to introduce something new to bring about continued improvement. That new thing can involve adding extra weight, doing additional repetitions (referred to as *reps*), adding new exercises, or shortening the amount of rest between sets. (If you lift a weight once, you've done one rep. If you lift a weight ten times in a row, that's one set of ten reps. And if you then take a slight break, and lift that weight ten more times, you've done two sets of ten reps each.)

In other words, you don't have to do a tremendous amount of exercise — you just have to ask your body to handle slightly more than it's used to, and keep doing that as you get into better shape.

For a balanced workout, you need to train all your major muscle groups:

- ✔ Chest
- ✔ Back
- ✔ Shoulders
- ✔ *Biceps* (the fronts of your upper arms)
- ✔ *Triceps* (the backs of your upper arms)
- ✔ Abdominals
- ✔ *Quadriceps* (your front thighs)
- ✔ *Hamstrings* (your rear thighs)
- ✔ Calves

Don't exercise the same muscle two days in a row. Muscles need time to recuperate and get stronger between weight-training sessions.

In this book, we don't have space to go into the proper technique and form you need to follow when doing weight training. So we recommend you work out with a personal trainer until you're comfortable performing the exercises on your own; find a weight-training DVD to work out with at home; or get a copy of *Weight Training For Dummies,* 3rd Edition, by Liz Neporent, Suzanne Schlosberg, and Shirley J. Archer (Wiley).

Staying Motivated

We'll let you in on a little secret: Nobody likes the effort it takes to exercise. What people love is the way they look and feel when they exercise regularly. When you feel good about yourself, sticking with your healthy lifestyle changes becomes easier.

Keeping extra weight off can be as challenging as losing it. Many things will tempt you to go back to your old habits. To keep the pounds off and retain your ideal weight, you'll discover that motivation is key.

Keep these suggestions in mind to help you stay on track and get you through the rough times:

- ✔ **Build on success.** Start with small goals that lead to larger goals.

- ✔ **Find an exercise partner or a class to help you stay interested.** You can cheer each other on, have company, and feel safer when you're outdoors.

- ✔ **If you aren't in the mood to exercise, think of how good you'll feel after your workout.**

- ✔ **Focus on new options that you'll have after you become healthy and fit.**

- ✔ **Reward yourself at special milestones — but not with food!** Nothing motivates like success.

- ✔ **Create variety in your routine.** This will help keep you from becoming bored with your program.

- ✔ **Hire a personal trainer.** Having someone else push you a bit can be all the motivation you need.

- ✔ **Remember that relapsing into old habits is not failing.** Every day is a new opportunity to get back on track!

- ✔ **Visualize yourself already at your goal.** Feel it, see it, believe it — because it can happen to you!

In addition to following all these tips, try keeping an exercise journal — a record of how much exercise you do — so you'll know what has been working for you and what hasn't.

Before starting, know your body weight. Weigh yourself first thing in the morning before eating breakfast, without clothes or wearing the same amount of clothing. Don't weigh yourself more than once a week. Record your weight in your exercise journal each time you do. Use a tape measure to measure your hip, waist, and neck. Measure around the widest point of each area. Use the same points consistently as you measure each part of your body. Record these measurements as well. You should take your measurements no more than once a month.

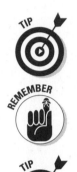

Take front and side pictures of yourself and keep them in your exercise journal. These pictures will be motivational when you look back and see how far you've come.

Keep in mind change happens slowly, and you may not see results for at least four weeks. Weight is not the only measurement of a healthy body. For example, as you burn fat and gain muscle, muscle weighs more than fat, so you may actually see a slight weight increase before you see a decrease.

Variety is the spice of life — and of exercise. Creating variety in your routine will prevent you from becoming bored, lead to greater enjoyment, and make it more likely that you'll stick with your program. As you exercise more often, over time your body will become accustomed to handling the same routine, and you'll no longer receive the maximum benefits of your efforts. You'll need to change your exercise plan in order to stimulate new growth.

Whatever you do, you have to keep adding to your challenges in order for it to bring about the kind of physical changes you're looking for. For aerobic activity, vary the speed, intensity, incline, or workload, depending on the activity you choose. For anaerobic exercise, increase the weights, sets, or reps, or change the order of your exercises.

Add some variety to your weekly routine by choosing different activities. For example, if your daily routine involves walking, try mixing it up by going swimming. Keep trying new sports, exercise DVDs, and gym machines until you find ones you truly enjoy. Then mix them up again!

Chapter 17

Enlisting Outside Help

In This Chapter

▶ Looking at your support-group options

▶ Making sure you get the follow-up care you need

Weight loss and weight maintenance are not easy even after surgery. You're still left with battling old eating issues, in addition to facing new problems such as dealing with new ways to eat, nausea, and maybe even hair loss. In this chapter, we give you suggestions of places to turn for help, no matter what challenges you face.

Joining a Support Group

Following weight loss surgery, it's very important that you don't try to go it alone. The surgery itself is just the first step in a long journey, and the road ahead will have ups and downs (both physical and emotional). Making sure you have someone to turn to when you need some help is essential to ensuring your success.

Support groups are great places to turn. In fact, studies have shown that those who attend support groups are more successful after weight loss surgery than those who don't. Having people traveling along with you will make your weight loss surgery journey easier.

You can find professionally led support groups (groups led by surgeons or by people who work on-staff in their practices), as well as peer-led support groups. There are also online support groups. Each type of group has its place and importance in your success.

Support groups can be a great help not only for you, but also for your family and friends. Feel free to take your spouse, significant other, friends, family members, and children. If you do take kids, be sure to take only those who can benefit from the experience and can sit quietly for two hours. Babies, toddlers, and very small children will only distract you and the group.

Local support groups

Depending on where you live, you may be able to find a variety of support groups in your area. In the following sections, we fill you in on the basic kinds of support groups you'll encounter.

Whether you're attending a surgeon-supported group or a patient-led group, keep in mind that there will be (or should be) different groups depending upon the type of surgery you've had. For example, it isn't a good idea to have gastric bypass, sleeve gastrectomy, and gastric banding patients in the same group, because gastric banding patients lose weight at a much slower rate and can be very discouraged when they hear about gastric bypass patients who are losing 20 pounds every month. In the end, gastric banding patients may lose as much as gastric bypass patients, but they'll just take a little longer to reach that goal. Surgeons also will separate duodenal-switch patients from other weight loss surgery patients because duodenal-switch patients can eat more food. And although a gastric bypass patient may be struggling getting down a cup of food and dealing with those issues, the duodenal-switch patient doesn't have those challenges. Finally, separating the groups is also important because a debate inevitably begins over which is the best surgery, with each group vigorously defending its choice.

Surgeon-supported groups

Most surgical practices have their own support groups. In fact, when you're choosing a surgeon, whether she has a support group is one of the factors you can use to decide. If the surgeon has a support group, odds are, she understands the importance of patient education (which is one of the keys to success after surgery). For more on choosing a surgeon, turn to Chapter 5.

Over and over, you'll hear that weight loss surgery is only a tool. The surgeon's role in your weight loss technically lasts the duration of the surgery, which is approximately two hours. It's up to you to use the tool you've been given to lose as much weight as you can and to find personal health. Attending support groups will help you to use that tool effectively.

Surgeon-supported groups are typically held once a month in a conference room of the hospital. The day of the month is fixed — for instance, a support group will meet the third Thursday of every month at 7 p.m. Meetings generally last two hours. There is no admission fee to attend support groups. Some practices charge an overall program fee, and the care and feeding of the support group is included; other practices financially support the group from the proceeds of the practice.

The group is generally led by the bariatric coordinator for the practice. Sometimes, a speaker will be brought in to talk to the group. You can expect to hear speakers on all kinds of topics, including plastic surgery, exercise, vitamins, digestive problems such as constipation and diarrhea, or body image. You may even get the chance to hear a celebrity speaker. Often, you'll be able to pick up educational handouts, such as articles of interest or recipes.

At other meetings, there will be no speaker, and the meetings will be open for questions and answers. Most often, the surgeon will attend part or all of the meeting. Other healthcare professionals associated with the practice (including nurses, dietitians, psychologists, or bariatricians) may attend as well. (See Chapter 5 for more on these key team members.)

Surgeon-supported groups are excellent places to have your questions answered by experts. If you're concerned about anything, these groups are your chance to have those concerns addressed. The groups don't replace a visit to your doctor, though. Follow-up care is equally important for long-term success.

Another important reason to attend a support group is to associate with others who are in the same position as you. You'll meet people who had surgery around the same time you did, and you can be great companions for each other. You can call each other and commiserate or join a gym together. You'll also meet people who had surgery years earlier. You can learn from their setbacks and be inspired by their successes.

Comparing notes on weight loss with the other patients at support-group meetings is only natural. Just remember that some people take more time to shed pounds, and others lose weight more rapidly. If you're not losing weight as fast as someone else is, don't feel as though you're failing. Everyone is different, and how rapidly you progress doesn't necessarily indicate how successful you'll ultimately be. Sometimes slow and steady truly does win the race.

If your surgeon doesn't have a support group, you may want to consider attending another local surgeon's support group. You may be accepted with open arms at these meetings — or you may not. It depends upon the dynamics of the group and the practice. Start by introducing yourself to the group leader and explaining where your surgery was performed and by whom. Be prepared to explain why your surgery was performed elsewhere. You also may want to consider calling the surgeon's office ahead of time to speak to the support-group leader instead of just showing up. You may be asked to pay a program fee to attend.

Support for each other

For me, support groups are the lifeline to remaining focused on the goal — first it was losing weight with my band, and now it's about using the groups to remain focused on my weight-loss maintenance. At my highest weight of 287, being involved with a support group began the direct education of what life would be like after surgery. I had contemplated surgery for several years and initially had gone to support groups with a friend of mine as her support person. I soon realized that surgery was the way to go for me, too, and because of the group I was able to feel secure in the decision I was making.

Throughout the weight-loss phase after my surgery, my support group was extremely important in continuing to encourage me through the ups and downs and keeping me engaged in the process. When my own resolve is waning, it helps me to focus on someone else and encourage them, knowing that not long ago, I was in that very place.

Years after my surgery, I still actively participate in several support groups, both in person and online, for the same reasons that I always have: Support groups are among the most important tools that I have to remain satisfied and successful in this difficult journey. We can never hear it enough: "Surgery is just a tool to help us lose weight." My add-on to that phrase is: "Support groups are the tool to help me continue to maintain my weight loss."

Tammy St. Clair
New York, New York

You should have a good reason for not having had your surgery performed by that surgeon. For example, perhaps your insurance wouldn't cover the surgery for that surgeon or hospital, or you just moved to the area.

Patient-led groups

If you live in an area where there aren't any surgeons performing weight loss surgery, and you and many other patients have had to travel a distance to have surgery, a patient-led support group may be your only option. These groups are excellent for peer-to-peer support even though there won't be a healthcare professional available to address your medical questions.

If you're thinking about starting a patient-led support group, find out how many people who live in your community are patients. Because of confidentiality laws, your surgeon can't give you names and addresses of patients. But he can do a mailing for you with your contact information, so other patients can get in touch with you. A local library or community hall is a good place to get together, because the meeting room will probably be free or have a nominal fee.

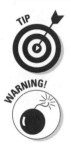

The Obesity Action Coalition offers support-group listings at `www.obesity action.org/advocacy/support-groups`.

A patient-led support group is not the ideal, because patients may start to rely on their peers for medical advice, which can be dangerous. At the very least, the person leading the group should be a healthcare professional who is a patient and has had weight loss surgery.

Whoever is leading the group should keep in contact with a surgeon's office. The regular support-group leader can supply handouts and suggestions for discussions. Encourage surgeons to attend at least every other month so the patients can ask nonemergency questions directly of a surgeon and get her expertise.

Online support groups

You may have various reasons for not wanting to attend a support group in person with other patients. You may have scheduling conflicts, or you may just not like groups. If so, an online support group may be a good fit for you. The advantage of an online support group is that it allows you to stay in touch on a daily basis with those who are going through what you're going through.

Participating in an online support group is definitely better than doing everything on your own, but an online support group doesn't compare to attending a surgeon-supported group, attended by healthcare professionals.

The majority of online support groups can be found at `http://groups. yahoo.com`. After registering with Yahoo!, type **weight loss surgery** in the search box, and you'll find hundreds of support groups you can join. You'll find a group for every problem, persuasion, and location. Here's just a sampling of some of the groups you can join:

- **OSSG_PreOps,** for those who haven't had surgery yet
- **OSSG-InsuranceHelp,** for those who need help with insurance approval
- **OSSG-Divorce**, for those who have had surgery and are going through or contemplating divorce
- **OSSG_Off_Track,** for those who are one year or more post-op and encountering difficulties
- **Vertical-Sleeve,** for those who have had sleeve gastrectomy
- **Bandsters,** for those who have had gastric banding surgery

✔ **DuodenalSwitch,** for people interested in learning about duodenal-switch surgery

✔ **OSSG-MinigastricBypass,** for patients who have had mini gastric bypass

Facebook is another great option for weight-loss groups. Some Facebook groups are sponsored by surgeons; others, by individuals who have had weight loss surgery, like WLS Private, a private Facebook group sponsored by author Barbara Thompson (to locate the group, go to www.facebook.com and type **WLS Private** in the search box).

Here are some other websites that can be of great help:

✔ **FitDay** (www.fitday.com): An online diet and fitness journal.

✔ **ObesityHelp** (www.obesityhelp.com): A popular site where you can get information by posing questions that are answered by other patients. For a fee, surgeons can list information about themselves.

✔ **Weight Loss Surgery Center** (www.wlscenter.com): The website of author Barbara Thompson. Here you can find extensive information and sign up for a free monthly e-newsletter.

Follow-Up Care

After weight loss surgery, you'll need to have continuing care from medical professionals, including your surgeon, even if you're feeling terrific. In the following sections, we fill you in on what you can expect.

With your surgeon

Your relationship with your surgeon should continue forever. You've gone through life-altering surgery, and you'll need to be monitored to see how the surgery is affecting you.

If you had gastric bypass, sleeve gastrectomy, or duodenal-switch surgery, you'll begin by meeting with your surgeon about seven to ten days after surgery for a general checkup. The first year, you'll go approximately five more times for checkups to see if you're having any problems and to answer any of your questions. After that, if you don't have any problems, you'll meet annually with your surgeon.

If you've had gastric banding surgery, you'll generally meet with the surgeon every month for the first year, every two or three months for the second year, and every six months thereafter. The band that forms your pouch will be tightened several times by injecting a saline solution through a port underneath your skin; the saline solution travels through a tube and goes into the ring or band. This injection of saline is done until the tightness is just right. As you lose weight, you may have a sense that the band is loosening, and fills are needed.

Regardless of the type of surgery you've had, one of the most important checks will be your blood work. Your surgeon knows what to look for and will order blood tests to look for nutritional deficiencies. These blood tests can mean the difference between being healthy and unhealthy. If a deficiency is found, you may just need one adjustment (such as an addition of a supplement or an increase in a food type) to remedy the problem.

Your surgeon also will check your weight to monitor how well you're doing. If you've regained some weight, your surgeon should have resources for you so that you can discover why. You can meet with a dietitian to discuss your diet, an exercise physiologist to discuss what exercises you can be doing, or a psychologist to discuss what mental barriers you may have that are causing you to regain.

With your primary-care physician

Your primary-care physician will continue to play an important role in your healthcare for annual physicals and monitoring your general health and medications. However, it's important that, for your surgical follow-up care, you see your surgeon on an annual basis long-term. You may have to meet with your primary-care physician rather than your surgeon for follow-up if your surgeon is located far from where you live.

Many primary-care physicians aren't knowledgeable about follow-up care of weight loss surgery patients and don't know exactly what to test for and what to look for. They may not be able to recognize a deficiency or know what tests to give to find a deficiency. Moreover, complications such as an internal hernia will be best recognized by your surgeon.

If you don't have access to your surgeon and your only follow-up care is through your primary-care physician, be sure that copies of your tests are sent to your surgeon to review. Encourage the physicians to communicate regarding your care.

With your bariatrician

A *bariatrician* is a physician trained in nutrition, metabolism, exercise physiology, and behavior modifications for patients with weight issues. Bariatricians have a wide range of options to offer their patients, including special diet and nutrition products, individualized exercise programs, suggestions for lifestyle changes, and prescription medications, if necessary. They can be helpful in your battle with obesity before and after surgery.

Some bariatricians are associated with a surgeon's practice, but most have their own practice. You can ask either your surgeon or your primary-care physician for a referral.

Part V
Changing Outside and In

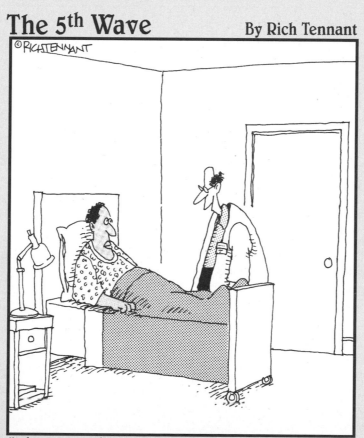

The 5th Wave — By Rich Tennant

"There are things to consider before electing a procedure to tighten your skin following weight loss surgery. For instance, would you like pleats?"

In this part . . .

You'll most likely hit rough spots along the way as your mind and body adjust to a totally new way of life and to your new physical reconfiguration. Some of these problems will be physical, such as hair loss, dumping syndrome, excess skin, and digestive problems. Other problems will be mental, as you try to deal with the incredibly drastic changes in your life. And the changes that you'll go through will affect all the relationships around you. Your family dynamics will be different because you're a much different person. In this part, we detail what to look out for and ways not only to cope but also to thrive.

Chapter 18

Avoiding Potential Pitfalls: Physical Challenges

. . . .

In This Chapter

▶ Identifying the likelihood of hair loss

▶ Delving into the causes of dumping syndrome

▶ Figuring out what's going on in your gastrointestinal system

▶ Looking into weight regain

. . . .

Your body will go through lots of physical changes after weight loss surgery. Some changes you may expect, and others may seem to come out of nowhere. In this chapter, we look at some of the more common physical changes within the first year after surgery, what they mean, and how you can deal with them.

Falling Asleep at the Wheel: Lack of Energy

You get home from the hospital and you're wiped out. After all, you did have major surgery. But how long should you expect this lack of energy to last? Any surgery stresses your body. As your body is healing, you'll feel fatigued. If you had gastric banding surgery, this fatigue may last for a week or two at most. If you had gastric bypass, sleeve gastrectomy, or duodenal switch surgery, the fatigue may last up to six or eight weeks.

You're eating and drinking a lot less. Your body is dealing with healing on fewer calories and, in some cases, *very* few calories. You also may be dehydrated because you can't get in the required amount of liquids.

Let your surgeon know that you're feeling fatigued. If you're beyond the two-to eight-week time frame, have your blood work checked. You may need vitamin B12 or you may be anemic. Your surgeon also will want to make sure you're getting enough protein in your diet.

Mouthing Off: Oral Problems

Your mouth is directly connected to your new stomach via your esophagus, so you'll experience some reactions to your surgery in your mouth.

Dry mouth

Right after any of the weight loss surgeries, your mouth will feel dry. This starts right after surgery and can persist for weeks. You probably won't be able to drink anything until you get an okay from your surgeon. You're also on pain medications that dry out your mouth. Over the next few days, as you start to drink and ease off the pain medications, you'll start to feel better — but dry mouth can be a recurring problem.

 Be sure to get at *least* 48 to 64 ounces of fluid every day, which may be a struggle — you just won't feel as though your new stomach is big enough to get all that fluid in. Drink as much as you possibly can. Eating sugar-free popsicles can help.

Bad breath

Yes, after weight loss surgery, your breath may smell. Bad breath may be a sign that you need to hydrate more. But if you're already drinking at least 64 ounces of fluids, a couple other issues may be the cause of your bad breath:

- ✔ **Food may not be emptying from your new stomach well.** Sometimes taking an antacid helps.

- ✔ **You may simply be forgetting to brush your teeth after meals.** Be sure to do so, focusing on the gums. Remember to brush your tongue as well.

- ✔ **You may be experiencing what's known as *ketotic breath*.** Ketotic breath is slightly sweet smelling and can occur as your body is losing weight, signifying the breakdown of proteins. A urinalysis will show ketones to confirm this diagnosis. Increase the protein in your diet to see if your breath improves.

Difficulty swallowing

After weight loss surgery, you'll find that food sometimes goes down and other times it doesn't. Watch how you eat — not too fast, not too big a bite, and be sure to chew, chew, chew!

If solids don't go down but liquids do, you may have a stricture or narrowing of the outlet of the stomach pouch to the intestines or your new "sleeved" stomach. If you have trouble with liquids, it may be a stricture but it could also be an ulcer. Call your surgeon to find out.

Getting something stuck in your new stomach is not fun. If you've eaten a piece of meat that seems to be stuck, mix some meat tenderizer in warm water and sip it slowly. The meat tenderizer will help to break down the meat so it can pass through. Don't wait too long if it looks like the new stomach is still plugged. Let your surgeon know before you get dehydrated. If you have food stuck for four hours, it's time to call the surgeon.

Nausea

When nausea occurs right after your surgery, it can be related to pain medications or even the anesthesia that you received. If it occurs in the weeks to months after your surgery, you may have an obstruction, an ulcer, or even low blood sugar:

- ✔ **Obstruction:** If you have an obstruction, you'll typically experience other symptoms, such as abdominal pain and vomiting. Your doctor may order abdominal X-rays and a CAT scan to diagnose a bowel obstruction.

- ✔ **Ulcer:** If you have an ulcer, it can be diagnosed with an upper endoscopy, which is done with a tube that is put down your throat. The ulcer can be treated with medication that decreases acid production in your new stomach.

- ✔ **Low blood sugar:** If you have low blood sugar, you may not be eating at regular times, and your caloric intake at meals can be very low. If the nausea is related to low blood sugar, eating a cracker usually will resolve the issue.

Peppermint has been long known to help with nausea and indigestion, which is why mints are commonly given after dinner. If you're having problems with nausea, try smelling peppermint oil, available at most drugstores, or drink some peppermint tea. Ginger, either fresh or as a tea, may help soothe your stomach as well.

Splitting Hairs: Hair Loss

As you lose weight, your body goes through all kinds of changes, and one of those changes involves hair loss. Hair loss can be tough to deal with. Your hair may be the one thing you really like about yourself. Also, it happens when you aren't nearly at your goal weight, so you aren't yet feeling good about yourself.

Your hair can come out in what looks like clumps. You may notice it in the shower drain and in your hair brush. You won't go bald, but there is a definite overall thinning effect. This usually occurs from the fourth month to the ninth month after weight loss surgery.

No one knows for sure why hair loss occurs, but it doesn't happen to everybody. After gastric banding, about 20 percent to 30 percent of patients experience hair loss of some sort. After gastric bypass, sleeve gastrectomy, and duodenal switch surgeries, the majority of patients have significant hair loss. It would be extremely unusual for someone to go bald. But if you have thinning hair to begin with, this amount of hair loss may be noticeable.

There is no cure for the hair loss — when your hair starts to fall out, you can't do much about it. In order to try to prevent hair loss, as soon as possible after the surgery make sure you're eating at least 60 grams of protein per day. You also may want to try a hair and nail vitamin or try taking zinc, vitamin E, or biotin. (Although none of these is scientifically proven to change the hair loss, they're worth a try.)

Good news! When your weight loss stabilizes, your hair loss slows down, and your hair does grow back. There is a theory that this hair loss occurs because of hormonal changes that occur with the weight loss, and that as the weight loss slows down, the hair loss slows down as well. Sometimes it grows back different than it was before — curly when before it was straight, for example!

Down in the Dumps: Dumping Syndrome

Dumping syndrome occurs when you eat something high in sugar or fat. It happens only to gastric bypass patients, but only in 30 percent to 40 percent of them. Here are the symptoms of dumping syndrome:

- Lightheadedness
- Sweating
- Nausea

> ✔ Heart palpitations
>
> ✔ Abdominal cramps
>
> ✔ Diarrhea

Basically, you feel horrible for about 20 to 60 minutes. And you don't want to repeat the experience — for at least a few months.

Dumping syndrome is a lifelong problem in only a small percentage of patients. Most patients who experience dumping syndrome after the surgery see a decrease in the severity of symptoms over time.

TECHNICAL STUFF

Why dumping syndrome occurs

With gastric bypass, chewed food, which is undigested, goes right from your mouth to the esophagus into your stomach pouch and directly into the small intestine. The difference from the normal anatomy is that the food enters the intestine very rapidly in gastric bypass, and it enters a portion of the intestine that isn't accustomed to having undigested food.

If you eat something high in sugar or fat, this causes excess fluid to rush to that area of the small intestine, and it makes you feel awful as dumping occurs.

Check the labels: A food or drink with less than 15 grams of sugar per serving shouldn't cause dumping. Some people have experienced dumping after eating fruit like watermelon or even a banana, as well as fatty foods like egg-drop soup.

Some sugars are more likely to cause dumping:

✔ Brown sugar

✔ Dextrose

✔ High-fructose corn syrup

✔ Honey

✔ Maple sugar

✔ Molasses

✔ Raw sugar

✔ Sucrose

Simple sugars that are normally well tolerated include

✔ Dextrin

✔ Fructose

✔ Galactose

✔ Glucose

✔ Invert sugar

✔ Lactose

✔ Maltose

✔ Sorbitol

✔ Sorghum

✔ Xylitol

Remember that "no sugar added" is not the same as "sugar free." You can still dump on no-sugar-added foods, because the food may have a lot of natural sugar, which may cause you problems. The best thing to do is look at the nutritional label and see how many grams of sugar are in each serving.

Many patients love dumping syndrome because it forces behavior modification. If you can't have foods high in sugar or fat because of a terrible reaction, how much easier is it to stay on your low-fat, low-sugar diet? Much! The downside of dumping is that even if you don't routinely eat sweets, having a small bite of birthday cake can cause dumping.

Somebody Call a Plumber: Bowel Problems

A common fallacy of weight loss surgery is that everyone has diarrhea. Well, the good news is, this isn't true. In the following sections, we fill you in on some of the not-so-fun bowel-related symptoms you may experience after weight loss surgery.

Constipation

Having a bowel movement every two to three days is normal. *Constipation* is defined as less than one bowel movement per week. (Most patients are used to having a bowel movement every day before surgery, so they think they're constipated when they really aren't.) Another hallmark of constipation is hard stools.

Constipation is probably the most common complaint after gastric banding, sleeve gastrectomy, and gastric bypass surgery, and it usually means you need to drink more. A minimum daily fluid intake is 48 ounces for women or 64 ounces for men. But the more you drink, the better off you are. Also, if you're taking a lot of narcotic pain medication, a side effect is constipation.

Another cause of constipation is a lack of fiber in your diet. When patients first start to eat, they tend to shy away from fiber because they're afraid something will get stuck. Prunes are a good option. If you're within four weeks of weight loss surgery, the prunes should be pureed. If you had gastric bypass, take a very small amount of prunes as a test dose, just in case you have dumping symptoms from the prunes. If prunes don't appeal to you, you may want to try a high-fiber cereal to help with constipation.

Suppositories, stool softeners, and enemas are always options to get things moving. Milk of magnesia is also a possibility with gastric banding and sleeve gastrectomy. If you've had gastric bypass surgery, let your surgeon know if you take milk of magnesia for constipation. Natural supplements like Senna are also options.

If constipation is a persistent problem, take added fiber — preferably the kind you drink rather than the pills. Benefiber, Citrucel, and Metamucil are all acceptable forms. All forms of fiber require additional water, because they work by absorbing water and making stools softer.

Diarrhea or loose stools

After gastric bypass and duodenal switch surgeries, loose stools are common.

What most patients think of as diarrhea, most surgeons would classify as loose stools. Surgeons classify true diarrhea as pure water.

With time, most stools become more formed in both gastric bypass and duodenal-switch patients. Initially, with gastric bypass, having two to four loose movements per day is normal; with duodenal switch, four to eight loose movements per day is normal. With time, one to two formed bowel movements per day are common with gastric bypass, and two to four formed bowel movements per day are common with duodenal switch. If you have a high-fat meal, you may have more bowel movements with duodenal switch and gastric bypass surgeries.

If you're experiencing pure water diarrhea, and you're having four to ten bowel movements or more a day, call your surgeon. You may be the victim of *gastroenteritis,* which is an inflammation of the lining of the intestines and stomach. If this is the case, staying hydrated is very important. You may require intravenous fluids. Signs of dehydration (which can be caused by diarrhea) can be a parched mouth, dark urine, and dry skin. This type of diarrhea has to be managed with close supervision by your surgeon, who may prescribe several different medications to try to counteract the frequency of the bowel movements. Although Imodium is commonly used, do not take it without your doctor's approval. Your surgeon also may want to make sure you don't have an infectious diarrhea known as *Clostridium difficile.*

Gas

Gas normally smells, but after weight loss surgery, your gas may be extremely foul smelling. If that's the case, first look at your dietary history and then contact your surgeon.

A few options are available. If your diet has changed to primarily meat, chicken, or dairy, this can affect the odor of your gas. Simplifying your diet may help decrease the odor. At least two dietary supplements are available online that help to decrease the odor of gas: Devrom and Nullo are designed as supplements for patients who have colostomies. These supplements help to deodorize your gas. Your surgeon may treat the odor with an antibiotic, but that's only done in a few cases.

In addition to your gas potentially being more foul smelling after weight loss surgery, you'll be more gassy than you were before. Because you're chewing your food so much more, as you chew more thoroughly, you'll be introducing more air into your system. In addition, you have to make more swallows to get a small mouthful of food down, which adds to the air you introduce into your gastrointestinal tract — all of which leads to more gas.

You'll also hear rumblings and gurglings from your intestines that seem like they must be dangerous. They usually aren't. The noise is just the air that you've swallowed making its way from your mouth through your body and out.

Warn your loved ones before the surgery. You'll soon get tired of saying "Excuse me."

Come Again? Weight Regain

Everyone who has weight loss surgery wants to believe that her weight loss is forever — and for some patients it is. But keeping all those pounds off takes a lot of work. Most patients experience a gradual weight regain. At five years after weight loss surgery, patients have kept off more than they have after ten years. That means that some of the patients have regained some of their weight. It's important to keep in mind that the studies represent averages, which means some people regain little to no weight, while others experience a slight regain, and still others regain a lot.

Your best defense is staying active and watching your diet. Sounds simple, but it's tough and it takes constant attention. Here are ways to help you succeed:

- **Meet with a dietitian.** She can provide you with a lot of support and specific guidance about your diet.
- **Keep a food journal and examine your eating habits.** You'll find no better tool to make you aware of everything that goes into your mouth.
- **Try not to slip into old routines, such as late-night eating, snacking, or grazing.**

If you do regain some weight, the first thing you may think is that you've failed at weight loss surgery. But you can get it under control — and you haven't failed.

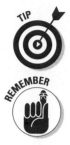

Your first step should be to book an appointment with your surgeon — no matter how long it's been since your surgery. Your surgeon will probably first do an upper GI series to make sure there isn't a physical reason for the weight regain. If nothing is physically awry, the surgeon will be able to tell you that the problem may be a result of your eating habits and exercise level.

Do your part, and get back to basics:

- ✔ Eat your protein first at any meal.
- ✔ Drink 64 ounces of water per day.
- ✔ Don't graze on food throughout the day.
- ✔ Exercise regularly.

Concentrate first on just stopping the weight gain. Get that under control first. Then after your weight is stable, you can work on losing the weight.

If you want to take off some or all of what you've regained, plan on sweating in the gym and doing some serious dieting. Just work on losing 5 percent of your weight and then increase your calories until your weight is stabilized. After your weight has been stable for a few months, work on losing another 5 percent. Take it in steps.

If you've regained all your weight, exercise and diet may not be options, and further surgery may be needed.

Low Blood Sugar: Hyperinsulinemic Hypoglycemia

Hypoglycemia is low blood sugar. *Hyperinsulinemic hypoglycemia* is low blood sugar caused by too much insulin.

When people have insulin resistance, their bodies produce insulin but their cells aren't recognizing the insulin, so the body has to produce even more insulin. After weight loss, these same cells can recognize insulin and better regulate blood sugar. After gastric bypass surgery, some patients have a surge of insulin when they eat carbohydrates, and their cells see too much insulin, which bottoms out their blood sugar.

Sometimes this syndrome is known as *late dumping*. The symptoms are similar to those seen in dumping (see "Down in the Dumps: Dumping Syndrome," earlier in this chapter). If you eat bread, for example, you can become ravenous an hour later. This condition can result in a constant hunger and weight regain.

In some patients, the symptoms of low blood sugar are so severe that they affect the brain; this condition is known as *neuroglycopenia*. The symptoms include forgetfulness, lightheadedness, excessive emotional reactions, and actually passing out. If you experience these symptoms, call your surgeon. You'll need to change your diet significantly, cutting out all simple carbohydrates (sometimes including fruit). You also may have to take special medications to help manage your hypoglycemia. Talk to your surgeon and the dietitian.

Chapter 19

Dealing with Post-Op Emotional Issues: What's Eating At You?

In This Chapter

▶ Understanding and dealing with hunger

▶ Recognizing and managing depression

▶ Avoiding your old eating patterns

▶ Setting yourself up to succeed

Chances are, before your surgery, food was something you turned to for all kinds of reasons other than hunger. You may have eaten when you were bored, tired, angry, happy, sad, lonely, or all of the above. Controlling your emotional responses to food can be the difference between success and failure following surgery.

In this chapter, we cover some common emotional, food-related challenges that weight loss surgery patients face. We also fill you in on some common behavioral obstacles that hinder success and show you how to overcome them.

Getting Your Head around Head Hunger

Everyone eats for many different reasons, and nutrition is usually last on the list. After weight loss surgery, you need to make nutrition your number-one priority. This means that, on most occasions, you choose foods that are healthy and nutritious for you.

Head hunger is hunger that's based more in emotions than in actual physical hunger. In this section, we help you figure out whether you're really hungry physically, or whether your hunger is coming from somewhere else. Then we give you some strategies to cope with head hunger.

Paying attention to whether you're really hungry

You'll naturally have different eating patterns at each stage of your recovery after weight loss surgery, and the type of surgery you've had makes a difference in what you'll experience. Here's what you can expect for each of the major types of surgery:

✓ **Gastric bypass:** Right after gastric bypass surgery, you may need to be on three meals a day and two snacks, because you can't get in the amount of protein necessary for the day any other way. As you progress farther out from surgery, you'll probably be on three meals a day, because you'll be able to get the nutrition you need within those three meals.

✓ **Gastric banding:** After gastric banding surgery, you'll probably be on three meals a day at the start. As you get adjusted with the band, that may decrease to two meals a day.

✓ **Sleeve gastrectomy:** After sleeve gastrectomy, you'll probably be on three meals a day.

✓ **Duodenal switch:** After duodenal switch, you may be on three meals and two snacks a day. This eating pattern may stay with you for a fairly long time, depending on how well you're able to take in the increased amounts of protein required.

Initially, after weight loss surgery, you may find you're less hungry. With time, some or all of your hunger returns. A meal may not satisfy you for as long as it used to. If you have a band, it may be time for an adjustment. If you have one of the other procedures, it may be time for some soul searching.

You're not alone if you often eat to escape from unpleasant situations. When the focus is on food, you don't have to be present in the current situation or feel the pain of not being able to trust or express yourself. Ask yourself whether you're hungry or whether you're

✓ Stressed

✓ Angry

✓ Bored

✓ Depressed

✓ Lonely

✓ Testing the limits of your surgery

✓ Feeling needy

If you've done all this soul searching and you find you really *are* hungry, ask yourself, "Can I make it to my next meal?" If you can, great. If you can't, find some healthy snacks that will help tide you over to your next meal.

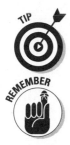

Be sure that, at each meal, you're eating until you feel full. Don't overeat to the point of stretching or throwing up, but be sure you're eating a full meal. This would normally include, for someone who is a year or more post-op, 3 to 4 ounces of protein, 1/2 cup of vegetables, and 1/4 cup of fruit or starch.

Don't drink anything with your meal, and eat your food slowly. If you eat too fast and don't chew your food well, you may get something stuck and confuse that feeling with fullness.

Each meal should last you at least four hours. If you're eating too little, you're leaving yourself vulnerable to getting hungry too soon and to snacking.

Fighting head hunger with some proven strategies

If you've asked yourself whether you're physically hungry and you decide that you aren't, you're experiencing *head hunger*. Head hunger may take the form of cravings (like for sweet or salty foods). You may not always be able to distinguish physical hunger from head hunger, but on the occasions that you *are* able to, what do you do?

Try to distance yourself from the reason that you're turning to food. Think of it as a timeout for yourself to allow you time to defuse. Instead of eating,

- ✔ Go for a walk.
- ✔ Get out of the kitchen.
- ✔ Drink lots of water.
- ✔ Walk up and down the stairs.
- ✔ Call someone who can help support you.
- ✔ If you're at work, walk around the office.
- ✔ Chew sugarless gum.
- ✔ Brush your teeth; brushing your teeth helps you stop eating late-night munchies.

To try to prevent head hunger, cut out all caffeine — caffeine can stimulate your appetite. Also, make rules, like no food after 9 p.m.

If you feel as though you just *have* to have something in your mouth, or that your mouth is always dry, don't start eating hard candies — sugar-free or not! These candies can become a bad habit. They have empty calories that you don't need.

If you can't control the head hunger, when you cave, cave with a little something rather than a lot of something. And remember, tomorrow is another day.

If you absolutely need to eat something, here are some healthy choices to always have around the house:

- ✔ A slice of low-fat deli ham or turkey
- ✔ Sugar-free Jell-O
- ✔ A protein drink made into a slushy
- ✔ Celery and carrot sticks
- ✔ Frozen grapes
- ✔ Hot herbal tea

Just remember that snacking on good things can lead to snacking on bad things, so be careful. If you recognize that you must eat more often, build the extra food into your day and write down everything you'll be eating, including the healthy snacks and the time that you'll eat them. This will keep you on track, and you'll come to understand the cycles of your own body.

Knowing when enough is enough

After weight loss surgery, you may still find yourself using food as a stress relief or a way to self-medicate. You may be thinking, "This is why I had to have surgery in the first place."

After weight loss surgery, some things are different. You don't have an endless capacity to eat. Because you now have a smaller stomach, your portions are restricted. Implement the better eating habits like eating for only 20 minutes. And try to look at what's making you turn to food. See what your triggers are and try to avoid them or get a better coping mechanism.

Ask friends and family for support when the head hunger is in high gear. Refusing food when you have head hunger is really difficult. If your support system just naturally offers you food out of habit or politeness, you end up battling not only your own demons, but also your family and friends. Talk to your family and friends and ask them to stop. Help them to understand that offering you food can put you on the road back to where you were before your surgery.

Conquering Depression

Many weight loss surgery patients experience depression after their surgery. If you feel depressed, it may not be any worse than the depression you felt before surgery, and you may not feel it every day. But it can happen, and you need to be prepared. In this section, we lead the way.

Identifying the symptoms of post-op depression

First, ask yourself if you were depressed before surgery. If the answer is yes, chances are, you're still going to be depressed after surgery — at least initially. As you lose weight, your depression may improve or even go away.

You may experience a new depression after surgery. This depression is related to all the changes your body is going through, as well as to your interactions with others. One of the signs of depression is fatigue, but if you're only a few weeks out from surgery, your fatigue may be just a natural part of recovering. Mood changes like anger and weepiness also can be signs of depression.

As you lose weight after your surgery, you may find yourself saying some of the following, all of which can lead to feelings of depression:

- ✔ I'm a failure because I had to have surgery to lose weight.
- ✔ I'm not losing enough weight.
- ✔ People are treating me differently now that I'm thinner. How can I trust them?
- ✔ I can't eat certain foods anymore and I hate that.
- ✔ I want to do more things, but my significant other doesn't.
- ✔ People are watching my weight loss. Are they waiting for me to fail?
- ✔ My life isn't perfect the way I thought it would be.
- ✔ I feel guilty that I'm still depressed even though I look better. I should feel grateful and happy that I was able to have this surgery.
- ✔ I miss being able to eat "big food."

If you're feeling down, talk to someone — your family, friends, surgeon, dietitian, counselor, or local or online weight loss surgery support group.

You're definitely not alone in how you feel. Many other patients go through the same thing. Your surgeon and her support staff will definitely have seen other patients who have gone through similar emotions and episodes. They have experience and will have some suggestions to help you.

Grieving over the loss of food

Food has been a good friend, support, strength, comfort, and love. Initially, after surgery, food won't be all these things to you, because you won't be able to get in the quantity of food that you could before surgery. Your taste for certain foods may have changed. Most of the rest of the time, if you overeat, you don't get a stuffed, comforting feeling, but an ugh, chest-pain feeling.

During the weeks and months after your surgery, you'll have days where you miss being able to use food for support. Realizing that a large amount of food will not make you feel better because you're physically unable to eat it is difficult. Realizing that you have to find some other way to make yourself feel better can be overwhelming.

Grieving over the loss of the role food once played in your life is a normal process, and most patients go through it. Try to remind yourself that your weight loss has resulted in significant health improvements. In time, your relationship with food will change, and you'll be happier (and healthier) because of that.

Dealing with Stress without Turning to Food

After your weight loss surgery, you need to find new ways to deal with stress — ways that have nothing to do with eating. In this section, we start by helping you figure out what's causing your stress. Then we give you some strategies for coping with stress in healthier ways.

Stress comes in many shapes and forms. If you're stressing out at work, is it because of your workload, your boss, or your co-workers? Is the stress directly related to your work, or is it related to social situations that arise at the water cooler? Is it the lunch hour that has you worked up? Is your weight loss the constant focus of attention? Do you still feel fatigued and unable to keep up with your work? Did you do too much before your surgery and now regret signing on for two jobs for the salary of one? Did you make yourself indispensable before your surgery and now wish you could take time off? Are you taking too much time off for medical follow-up, and is that a problem?

Stress also can come from family and friends. Is your weight loss causing problems in your marriage? Is your spouse jealous of new attention you may be getting? Are your friends saying you've changed since you lost weight? Are they hinting that they want the "old you" back? Do you find that you want to do new things and you have no one to do them with?

The first step in tackling stress is figuring out exactly what's causing it. Keep a diary of your daily activities to help you identify your most significant triggers for stress. Every time you get stressed out, write down what specifically made you feel stressed. Over time, you may notice a trend. When you feel stressed and ready to reach for something to eat, take a deep breath and analyze what caused that reaction.

After you figure out what causes you to stress out, the trick is to *decrease* the stress and not avoid it. If you've decreased your stress triggers, you'll be less likely to start snacking. For example, if your stress is related to your workload, you may be able to delegate part of your work to someone in your department. If that isn't possible, and you're expected to put in more than an eight-hour day, talk with your boss. Unfortunately, if you're expected to put in as many hours as it takes to get the job done, you may have to look around for another job. Set limits for yourself. Try to figure out what exactly you can accomplish in a day and try to stick to a schedule.

If your stress is related to social situations at work, confront the issue head on and discuss the problem with your supervisors or co-workers. If it's food-related, bring your own lunch so you won't throw up in front of the entire office. If you frequently have to entertain clients, call ahead to the restaurant and make sure the chef will make something you'll be able to tolerate. And if your clients wonder why you aren't eating a lot, have a ready answer like, "I had a big breakfast," "I'm on a diet," or "I'm not feeling well."

Stress from family and friends is an entirely different matter. You can't quit your family and friends — in most cases, at least. But you can be pretty direct with them. Try telling them exactly what's making you stressed and see which of your behaviors they're not so happy about. (After all, unless you're perfect, odds are you're stressing them out from time to time, too!) Sometimes just talking through your feelings is enough to resolve them. If talking doesn't seem to do the trick, see if you can get some family counseling to help everyone work through the problem.

If you find yourself turning to food in times of stress, try these tips:

- ✔ **Remove yourself from the stressful situation.** Try to get a little perspective, if you can.

- ✔ **Walk away from the food or the stress.** Exercise is a great stress reliever!

- ✔ **Focus on the success you've had with your weight loss.** This will help you strengthen your resolve not to succumb to stress eating.

- ✔ **Try to make healthy choices if you do need to eat.**

- ✔ **Try relaxation techniques.** If you don't know any, try enrolling in a yoga class at your local YMCA or community college. Or check out *Relaxation For Dummies,* by Shamash Alidina (Wiley), which comes with an audio CD with relaxation exercises you can follow.

- ✔ **Chew sugarless gum to keep yourself from turning to food.** Just keep in mind that chewing gum may make you more gassy.

Knowing What to Do If You're Having Trouble with Success

All you've ever wanted was to be less heavy. Now you're losing weight and other feelings come into play. What's it all about? In the following sections, we fill you in on some of the common emotional traps that you may fall into after weight loss surgery.

Feeling fragile: Buoying yourself with the support you need

As you lose weight, you gain self-esteem, become more outgoing, and feel more independent. But one look, one harsh word, or one unkind gesture can have you running for the hills. One step forward can easily turn into ten steps back. You're stepping lightly into new territory — whether it's into the dating scene or even within your existing relationships.

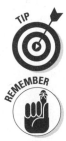

You may look for acknowledgement from those you love in what you've accomplished — and you may not get it. If this happens, look to your support structure or find a new one, such as an online or local support group. Discuss what you're going through with your surgeon or someone on his staff.

They aren't going to be able to solve any issues for you, but they'll listen, and you may get a helpful suggestion. Continuing on your road to improved self-esteem is the important thing.

Feeling fragile or insecure in the beginning is totally normal. Surround yourself with people who understand what you're going through and enjoy the ride — even if it's bumpy at times.

Feeling diminished: Avoiding negative people and negative thinking

You had surgery to lose weight, and in your post-op journey, you'll likely encounter people who will try to diminish your success by saying you took the easy way out. The person saying that may even be you. If you find yourself diminishing your successes, remember that nothing was really easy. You took a lot of risks and did a lot of work to relearn eating behaviors.

Some people may try to minimize the changes you've made by saying nothing's changed — you may have lost weight, but you may still be fat. These are the people you want to distance yourself from. They're hurtful, and they're wrong.

You have to lose only 10 percent to 15 percent of your total body weight to have significant improvements in your health. That's a change! Celebrate the positive. Don't let other people keep you down.

Feeling smaller: Recognizing that size doesn't equal power

Losing weight means that you're smaller in size — and smaller may mean less powerful to you. You may feel small, weak, and powerless. These feelings may lead you to try to regain some weight to become big and strong again.

Your power doesn't come from your physical size. Having lost weight, you're actually even more powerful than you were before — you've set a goal, made a commitment, worked hard, and improved your health. If that's not powerful, we don't know what is!

Feeling scared: Facing your fears

Part of your weight loss recovery involves fear — fear that you'll fail, fear that the weight loss will stop too soon, fear that the weight will all come back. These fears are very common after surgery. Fears are part of the reason you may not see the weight loss changes in the mirror initially — you're afraid to believe it because you know what the natural history of your diets has been: Lose some and gain back more.

Don't give up. No matter how far out you are from surgery, you still have control over what you eat and how active you are. True, there is a window of opportunity for weight loss, but when you regain some weight, you can create your own window to lose.

Breaking Old Habits

After your weight loss surgery, you'll probably resort to some old habits. After all, old habits die hard. They only go away after you've spent a long time working on them. Although you now have your surgical tool to help you, you break old habits by taking one step at a time.

In the following sections, we take a look at some of the old habits you may have and help you find ways to break them.

Grazing

Grazing (snacking on food all day long) is definitely something you have to stop right away after surgery. If you're getting all your nutrition in your meals, you shouldn't be grazing all day.

In order to stop grazing, you have to get rid of the things you like to graze on and you have to stay out of the kitchen. Try taking sips of water or Crystal Light when you get those urges. Don't sit in front of the TV and munch on food. Go to online support groups or head out for a walk.

Cravings

After surgery, you'll still have cravings and, in some cases, you start to crave new things. You may crave crunchy foods or sweet ones. Because weight loss is about taking in fewer calories than you burn, you can't give in to the cravings all the time. However, every once in a while, you can indulge — just try to limit the damage. For example, have one piece of chocolate instead of the whole candy bar. The good news: Controlling your portions is much easier after weight loss surgery.

Figuring out how to control cravings is important if you want to achieve your goals. In your food journal, document when and where you had a craving and what food you craved. See if you can identify specific people, emotions, places, and situations. Sometimes just acknowledging that you're experiencing a craving gives you the control you need to resist eating. But the ultimate goal is to reduce cravings by breaking the link to what triggered the craving in the first place.

Bingeing

Bingeing (eating without being able to control yourself) is about emotional needs more than a sense of physical hunger.

You can get violently ill from bingeing if you eat fast enough. Your new stomach can hold only so much — so you'll either throw up from eating too much or cause your esophagus to dilate from having too much food down there. Either way, causing damage to your new stomach or esophagus is no way to deal with your emotions.

Bingeing can be treated only if you treat the reason why you're bingeing in the first place. Identify the stress and make changes. Bingeing behavior is not healthy.

Testing the Limits

Periodically, you may find yourself lapsing either into old behaviors or behaviors you know aren't good for the long term. What's going on? You're testing the limits of what your weight loss surgery can do. You're seeing exactly how hard you have to work to either maintain or continue to lose.

You may notice that you're eating more at one sitting, or in between meals, or both. You tell your surgeon, "I'm able to eat more." Your surgeon asks, "Yeah, but are you hungry?" And the answer usually is no. You're realizing that you can eat at different times of the day and you're able to get in a certain quantity of food throughout the day.

This is a battle between your new stomach and your eyes. How much can you eat and still manage to lose weight or maintain your weight? This amount will change as you get farther away from surgery. *Remember:* As you lose weight, your body becomes more efficient and burns fewer calories. If you give in to your eyes and continue to eat bigger portions or more meals per day, you'll start to regain some of the weight.

Most patients say that at some point after the surgery, they start to crave chocolate or other sweets. Why? To some degree, there is a part of you that doesn't want you to succeed. Another part of you is waiting for the other shoe to drop — you're waiting for that point in recovery where your weight starts piling back on. The truth is, if you're making healthy food choices on most days and being reasonably active, you'll be able to maintain your weight. Succumbing to poor eating behaviors will only sabotage your weight loss.

Keep in mind that there is no reason you need to have chocolate every day. But every once in a while, if you want to have a piece (not the whole bar), go ahead.

Saboteurs take the form of family, friends, and, unfortunately, yourself. Weight loss surgery is a journey that really brings you in touch with who you are, what your fears are, and who your friends are. It brings into focus how people perceive you and how your weight impacts your relationships. Sometimes testing the limits is a form of self-sabotage.

Empower yourself and believe that you can be successful in this one area of your life that has eluded you in the past. Try to figure out if something is holding you back. Will a particular relationship be poorly affected by your weight loss? Or is this about your not loving yourself enough to succeed? Think about it, and make the changes that will allow you to win!

Chapter 20

Me, Myself, and I: Your Relationship with Yourself

After weight loss surgery, you still may think of yourself as the size you used to be — your sense of yourself may lag behind the reality. In this chapter, we discuss how your perceptions of yourself affect self-esteem. We help you adjust your body image to fit your new body — and we guide you through the changes you'll need to make as you lose weight.

Self-Esteem: Your Greatest Asset

We live in a society that values "thin." Look at any magazine and you'll see article after article on dieting. The models in these magazines are thin, often to the point of anorexia. Even though the average dress size is 14, the models are dressed in size 0.

Unless you live in a vacuum, you can't help but get many of your ideas of ideal size from the media. You can easily end up measuring your own self-worth by an unattainable and unhealthy standard.

You may have spent your adult life dieting to reach that size 0 and failed over and over again. Losing and regaining weight can really wreak havoc on your sense of self-worth.

Everyone has some kind of failure in his life. Some people have a job they dislike; others have financial problems; and still others have trouble with a child. People can choose to keep those failures private if they want. But when you fail in controlling your weight, that failure is out there for everyone to see. Your failure with your weight is a very public thing — everyone knows it, and you've probably suffered because of that.

Many people who are severely obese started battling weight when they were children. They've endured teasing by other children and sometimes being nagged by their parents.

Feeling like a failure is not new to many severely obese people. Is it any wonder that, after surgery, many people have a hard time believing that they'll maintain that weight loss and that they deserve the healthier, happier life that goes along with it?

In this section, we focus on common self-esteem issues and give you suggestions for how to overcome them.

Facing the possibility of success

Yes, you read that right. Sometimes the thought of succeeding — of reaching your weight loss goal — can be terrifying. Some people are surprised to find that they start to feel very vulnerable as they lose weight. They feel smaller and less powerful than they did when they were bigger and had that extra weight surrounding them as a barrier.

Do you have a weight at which you feel "safe," a weight at which you feel comfortable with yourself and feel healthy? This weight may not be your lowest weight. If this feeling of safety is very strong, you may find yourself gaining weight until you reach that "safe" weight.

In fact, this feeling of safety is sometimes why people regain weight after surgery. Even though they may be unhappy about the regain, the higher weight may just "fit" them better.

If you've regained weight after surgery, or if you've stopped losing at a weight that's higher than your original goal, the most important thing to consider is whether this weight is within the normal weight range on the BMI chart. If it is, there's absolutely nothing wrong with staying at this weight. You may want to stay at this weight permanently, or you may want to stay at it for a while, until you're comfortable with losing a little more.

If your "safe" weight is in the upper ranges of the "overweight" range on the BMI chart or into the "obese" ranges, that's a problem. If your "safe" weight puts you in an unhealthy zone, think about why you feel uncomfortable with your weight loss. If you have negative feelings about the success you've achieved, you may want to look out for some warning signs in yourself:

- Do you feel guilty about your success? Do you feel that you don't deserve to be thin?

- Are you viewing your body in a negative way all the time?

- Do you sometimes wish you hadn't lost weight?

- Are you having so many problems with excess skin that you hate your body and wish you would regain the weight to fill in the sags?

- Does being thinner make you feel weak and vulnerable?

- Being thinner, do you feel that people get too close to you?

- Do you feel very uncomfortable because people are noticing you more and are attracted to you?

- Do you feel disappointed because being thin hasn't taken away all your problems?

If you answer yes to these questions, talk to a psychologist or counselor about what you're feeling. (Your surgeon should be able to direct you to a psychologist who works with weight loss surgery patients.) These questions are important ones to ask yourself, and they're worth talking about at support-group meetings and with the support staff at your surgeon's practice.

Get outta my space!

Being smaller also means that you take up less space. As your physical space shrinks, so does what is referred to as your *personal space.* Personal space is that area around you that you need between yourself and others. When other people enter your personal space, you feel crowded.

We get a sense of where someone else's personal space is by that person's size. As you grow smaller, so does your personal space. If you don't have an accurate sense of your size, your sense of your own personal space is off-kilter. You may feel that people are getting too close to you, and that may make you feel very uncomfortable. As you become more accustomed to your true size, those feelings will lessen. Just give yourself time and know that your feelings are perfectly normal.

Many people experience these feelings, so don't think for a minute that you're alone or that something is wrong with you for feeling this way. Talking to other people who've gone through what you're going through, or talking to a therapist who's skilled in helping weight loss surgery patients, can help you work through your fears and insecurities.

Believing in yourself

If you've failed with dieting over and over (a prerequisite for having weight loss surgery in the first place), you may have trouble believing that this time it's really going to work. Only time and your own success will convince you of that. As the pounds disappear and you're able to sustain that weight loss, the belief will start to kick in.

Even if you regain a few pounds, you've still accomplished something wonderful!

Taking on new challenges

As you're losing weight after surgery, you'll find that you have better health and an improved way of life. You'll be able to do many things you've never been able to do or haven't done in a long time. If you aren't yet happy with the way your body looks, concentrate on the many things you're able to do.

Start by making a list of ways in which your life has improved. For example, you may be able to say

- I'm off my medications.
- I'm able to run up a flight of stairs without feeling like I'm going to die.
- I can wear a pair of slacks with a belt and tuck in my top.
- I can get down on the floor and play with my children and get back up again.
- I can see my toenails — and even paint them.
- I can take a bath and have water on both sides of my body.
- I can ride the bus or train and fit in one seat.
- I can cross my legs.

ANECDOTE

A journey to self-esteem

After so many years of being unable to keep weight off, I found it difficult to believe that my weight loss surgery would work. I also had to deal with guilt as I was losing. When people would congratulate me on losing weight, I felt like a cheater and was compelled to tell them that it wasn't really me who was losing the weight — I owed it all to gastric bypass surgery. Every time I saw an overweight person, I felt guilty that I had this wonderful opportunity that she may not have.

It wasn't until the middle of the third year that I truly started to feel confident in my ability to maintain my weight loss. Oddly enough, it began when I started to put weight on.

Due to a very stressful year, I had stopped exercising and had started eating more and more junk food. At first, I panicked. Here comes failure . . . again. Then I reminded myself that I still had this wonderful "tool." What would happen if I simply started exercising again and corrected my eating? That's exactly what I did, and the weight began to come off. I finally felt in control and that it was me doing it and not just the surgery!

It wasn't only losing weight that made my self-esteem climb. Every time I walk or exercise and can really feel my body respond, my self-esteem climbs even higher. It's been a long journey and perhaps I have more challenges in store, but now I know that I can do it! Now I am a "loser" — but in the best possible way.

Kalli Cagle
Pinellas Park, Florida

Then set some goals you'd like to accomplish. Write down these goals and post them where you can see them often. Here are some goals you may want to tackle:

- ✔ Go to an amusement park with your children and ride all the rides.
- ✔ Get down in the dirt and plant a garden.
- ✔ Go hiking.
- ✔ Go shopping without getting totally worn out.
- ✔ Exercise for a minimum of 30 minutes and enjoy it.
- ✔ Learn a new sport that you never thought you could do.
- ✔ Run for a local government or school office.
- ✔ Have a family portrait taken.
- ✔ Take a vacation in an airplane without using an extender on the seat belt.
- ✔ Run a 5K race.

As you achieve each goal, cross it off — doing what you've set out to do will give you a great sense of accomplishment! Challenge yourself to do things you never thought possible.

Body Image: Who Is That Person in the Mirror?

Close your eyes and try to get a mental picture of yourself. What you see is your *body image*. Body image is also how you think others see you and how comfortable you are with yourself.

With your body changing so rapidly, your mind may need a while to catch up with reality. You probably see yourself as larger than you really are, and it may be years before you realize just what you look like to the world.

You may have reached a number that you would have considered "successful" before your surgery, but you still don't feel good about yourself. The BMI chart may say that your weight is in the normal range, but you still see yourself as very overweight. You may walk through a door sideways as if you're too large to fit through the door walking straight through it. You may avoid going through turnstiles thinking you won't fit, or still think you need to ask for a table rather than a booth at a restaurant. If you find yourself in these or similar situations, you may have a problem with your body image.

Many weight loss surgery patients have the experience of not recognizing themselves in the mirror. You may be walking down a street and catch a glimpse of yourself in a store window and not realize that the person you're seeing is you.

Discovering that the image looks far better than you expect can be fun, but it also can be disconcerting. Not recognizing yourself can make you feel as though you've lost your identity. It may even mentally send you in search of that identity — some people find that the way to regain their identity is to regain weight. As unhappy as they were with that overweight person, at least they knew who they were. They don't know this new image, and that can be very frightening.

When you're very unhappy with the way you look and have an incorrect idea of what you look like, psychologists call this *body-image disturbance*. You think you look far worse than you really do. On its website, the Renfrew Center, an organization that focuses on women's mental-health issues (especially eating disorders), offers tips for identifying if you may have a body-image disturbance. Check out www.renfrew.org/body-quiz.asp for its list of questions.

When others tell you to stop losing weight

Your family and friends think of you in a certain way. And that certain way may be that you're heavy. That's their image of you, especially if you've been heavy for a number of years.

Many people look very healthy when they're heavy. Your chubby cheeks may have exuded health, even if the weight was taking a physical toll. And for those in your support system who are older and still haunted by the hardships of the Great Depression or are of an ethnic origin that values being large and strong, an over-weight body also may signify health. To them, anything is better than starving, and losing weight may be a negative.

As you lose weight so rapidly, you may hear warnings from people that you're losing too much weight. They may tell you this for a number of reasons:

✔ **If you aren't eating adequate protein or drinking enough water, your skin can appear very old, and they may be reacting to that.** Your skin may sag a lot, and you may look haggard. Be sure you're eating 60 grams of protein daily and drinking 64 ounces of water. *Remember:* This physical appearance of your skin is temporary and will improve with time.

✔ **Many people don't like change.** You'll be changing so rapidly that the problem is with them not you. They're just having a problem adjusting to your new form.

✔ **If you've always been the largest person in your circle of friends or family, someone else is going to have to take your place as the largest person.** Chances are, that person won't like it. He may have taken comfort in the fact that at least he wasn't as big as you. If you're getting smaller than he is, he may start to tell you that you're losing too much weight.

✔ **You may be losing too much weight.** Check your BMI (see Chapter 14) to see if you're in the normal weight range or the under-weight range. If you're underweight, schedule an appointment with your doctor.

What can you do to appreciate yourself and how far you've come? Here are some suggestions:

✔ **Take a good look at yourself in the mirror.** Just stare for a long time and appreciate that you've lived and loved and that your body reflects the good and the bad that you've been through. Understand that weight loss surgery won't erase the years, but it will give you many health and life benefits.

✔ **Look at your before pictures.** You may not remember what you looked like before you had your surgery. Have pictures taken now and compare the before and after pictures. This strategy is more effective than comparing the before pictures with a mental image, because you can look at the two side by side.

✔ Exercise and appreciate all the movements that your body can now do that it couldn't do before.

✔ Make a list of all the wonderful and unique things that make you special.

✔ Don't talk about dieting and your weight all the time. Direct your focus elsewhere.

Revamping Your Wardrobe

The saying that "Clothes make the person" is true. People put a lot of emphasis on their clothes, so as your body is changing so rapidly, you may find yourself scrambling to adjust to a shrinking size and a change in style. In this section, we let you know what you can expect when it comes to the clothes you wear.

Losing those comfort clothes

Don't you just love your comfort clothes? They're the ones you put on when you get home from work. They're the ones that make you feel really good, the ones you don't even have to think about whether they match or not. They're never too small. They never pinch or tug. They just hang there, completely forgiving. And you love them.

After surgery, you'll reach a point when your comfort clothes will be too large for you, and that can be devastating. Your comfort clothes will be so large that you'll be tripping over them, or they'll fall off.

When you reach that point, think about what you really like about your comfort clothes and try to duplicate that feel in new clothes. Look in the lower-priced stores or even in thrift shops for something smaller, but loose, soft, and comfortable. At first, these new clothes won't feel like a very good replacement — but in time, you'll feel just as comfortable in them as you did in your old comfort clothes.

Working around your excess skin

After you've lost weight, you may be left with a lot of excess skin that will have an impact upon the clothes you can wear. If you have those large "bat wings" (skin hanging down on your upper arms), your arms may not fit into the sleeves of a top that otherwise fits you just right. You may have to wear sizes too large for you to accommodate your loose skin.

If plastic surgery is out of the question, take your clothes to a tailor so you can be fitted properly. Or take a sewing course and learn to do your own alterations. If you have a new, smaller body, you don't want to hide it under clothes far too large for you.

Keeping up with your ever-shrinking body

So, what are you supposed to wear on the journey down to your ideal weight? You probably have clothes in your closet that you've long been hoping to fit into one day. You may have been through many sizes and still have those smaller clothes in your closet. Maybe you wore them for a brief time, wore them many years ago, or bought them as incentive to lose weight. Whatever the reason, you may have clothes ranging from size 10 to size 24.

You've been praying for the day when you could get back into those smaller sizes. Well, that day is here! But you may find that the clothes you had been holding on to in hopes of fitting into one day are now hopelessly out of date.

Many people find that they're losing weight so rapidly and they're going through sizes so fast that they can't keep up. The idea of getting clothes that fit when you may be in that size for only a brief period is discouraging. Here are some tips for dealing with those changing size requirements when you're losing weight so quickly:

- ✔ **Check out exactly what you have in your closet first.** When going through your closet, sort your clothes by size from the largest to smallest so you know exactly what you have. Take an inventory, so you don't go out shopping for a size that you already own.

- ✔ **Actually try on your old clothes.** You may surprise yourself that you can fit into a size you only dreamed about or saw only briefly, many years ago.

  Sizes today are not the same as sizes years ago. If you have a size 16 that is only a year or two old and one that is decades old, those two pieces of clothing will fit you differently. Manufacturers are making sizes much larger than they did years ago. So, if you try on an old version of a size and it doesn't fit, you may fit into a newer version of that same size.

- ✔ **Check with your support group to see if it has clothing exchanges where members bring in clothes that no longer fit them.** Take

advantage of these and get some smaller sizes that you'll wear only a
month or two. If your support group doesn't do a clothing exchange,
organize one yourself.

✔ **Ask family members or friends to help you.** Determine what your
size is and ask whether anyone has clothes that you can borrow for a
little while.

✔ **Shop in a consignment or secondhand shop or at your local Goodwill.**
They often have new or gently used clothes for a fraction of the cost.
Many people donate to Goodwill perfectly good clothes that you can add
to your wardrobe; you'll be helping a good cause at the same time.

✔ **Buy a few pieces of clothing that are flexible and forgiving and that
will shrink with you as you're losing weight.** A spandex and Lycra combination works well for this. It drapes well but doesn't cling.

✔ **Whatever you do, don't wear clothes that are too large for you.** They'll
make you look baggy and unattractive. Get out of those big clothes and
into something that fits.

Costume change

One thing that really blew my mind during the weight-loss process was how my wardrobe was affected — and thus, my wallet! As the weight came off, buying smaller and smaller sizes of jeans became a necessity, and quite frequently.

At any given time, I usually had only one, or two if I was lucky, pairs of jeans that actually fit, along with a handful of blouses that were size-appropriate. Plus-size clothing that I had spent hundreds, maybe thousands, of dollars on in the past quickly became unwearable.

When I reached my goal weight, hauling out all my old "fat" clothes to sell at a garage sale was quite cathartic. Many plus-size ladies were absolutely *thrilled* to find such a huge selection of reputable clothing in a range of about eight different sizes — not to mention the unbeliev-able deal they were getting: $1 for a sweater that originally cost me $45!

More than anything, though, it was like losing weight all over again to get out from under all of those old, big clothes.

My next "problem" became one of building a new wardrobe for myself, basically from scratch! I'm talking winter *and* summer clothes — shirts, pants, shorts, skirts, dresses, swimwear, pajamas . . . the list was endless!

For the first time in my life, I was bursting with excitement at the thought of shopping for hours on end just to buy myself some new clothes. Before my surgery, shopping had been a sad, confidence-destroying experience where my main concern for a purchase was: Does it cam-ouflage my huge stomach well enough?

My closet is now full of size-small clothing, and it's overwhelming to look back at the journey that has brought me to this point.

Amanda Foxworth
Fishers, Indiana

Figuring out where to shop

You've worked your way down through the sizes in the plus-size stores. But when you find that those are now too big, you need to face the intimidating world of clothing stores that sell regular sizes.

After years of being made to feel as though you don't belong in department stores, going into these stores can be an ordeal. You may still see yourself as very heavy. But the size that may be right for you can be found only in a regular store. You may worry that the salespeople will look at you as though you're there to buy a gift or gently ask if you're lost. Will they assume that you got turned around and wandered out of the plus-size department?

And what stores should you go into? Where are the styles and sizes to be found now? You know where to park your car in the mall lot when you shop at the plus-size stores. Where will you park and what direction will you head now? What regular-size stores carry the style of clothes that you like? These ideas may keep you in clothes far too large for too long because the whole ordeal is too much for you to deal with.

Here are some tips for navigating around this strange new fashion world:

- **Ask a friend who shops in regular-size stores and who wears clothes that you like where she gets her clothes.** If she shops in a department store, ask her not only the name of the store, but the floor, the department, and where the department is located.

- **Ask a friend to take you shopping.** Explain to her that you're having problems knowing where to shop and ask her to give you a tour. Make a day of it and buy her lunch.

- **Take advantage of personal-shopper services offered by some department stores.** Personal shoppers are employees of the department store, and their job is to help people shop. Ask at the customer-service desk if the store has that service.

- **Don't wait until you need clothes for a special occasion.** Do your research ahead of time.

- **Buy clothes that show off rather than hide your new body.** You don't have to wear dresses with long jackets anymore. Try tucking your shirt into your skirt or pants. You probably now have a waist, so show it off!

The first time you go into a regular department store and try on something and it not only easily clears your hips but you have to shout out, "Excuse me, but do you have this in a smaller size?" is a thrilling day. Enjoy every minute of it. You've earned it!

Chapter 21

Working At Relationships: Family, Friends, and Everyone in Between

• •

In This Chapter

▶ Recognizing how your surgery affects the people you love

▶ Considering kids and pregnancy

▶ Getting back into the dating scene after surgery

▶ Factoring in your friends

• •

*A*fter weight loss surgery, your body goes through rapid changes, and it's only natural that your family and friends will react to them — some positively and some negatively. Many of your friends and family will applaud and encourage you every step of the way; others won't be as helpful. You can't really be sure ahead of time how anyone will respond.

Sit back, take a deep breath, and read on for ways to survive relationships after surgery — whether they're relationships you've had for a long time (with family and friends) or ones you'd like to add to your life (with new partners and children). In this chapter, we help you see the role that others play in your weight loss surgery journey and what you can do to give your relationships the best chance for success.

Helping Your Marriage Weather the Storm

Under the best of circumstances, marriage is full of challenges. When one spouse is going through the kind of dramatic changes that weight loss surgery brings, those challenges only increase in number. Keeping a relationship humming and healthy during such a time of turmoil and change is more than many relationships can withstand. But for some relationships, the positive changes that weight loss surgery brings translate into positive changes in the relationship.

In the following sections, we fill you in on some of the positives and negatives you may see in your marriage after weight loss surgery. We also give you some tips for ways to keep your marriage going strong.

The good and bad news about weight loss surgery and marriage

Weight loss surgery brings with it all kinds of change — not only for the person having the surgery, but for the spouse. As with most things in life, the news isn't all good or all bad — your marriage may face some challenges at the same time that it sees significant rewards. In the following sections, we give you an idea of what to expect.

The good news

Weight loss surgery can make good marriages better. As you lose weight and feel healthier, your self-esteem soars. You start to like the way you look. You feel proud that you're finally able to lose weight, something you've failed at in the past. You catch a glimpse of yourself in a mirror and you start to like what you see. You may even find yourself taking a second look and thinking, "Hey, I look *good!*" When you like yourself more, you're able to love those around you even more, because you recognize that you have a lot to offer.

Before your surgery, you may have suffered from health problems. When you didn't feel well, you may have been cranky. And your spouse may have gotten the brunt of your bad mood — sometimes over nothing at all. But as you start to lose weight and your health problems start to improve or even disappear, your mood will improve — and your spouse will notice the difference.

After your weight loss surgery, you'll have a renewed sense of energy. You can be more active with your spouse and enjoy going out. You'll no longer be afraid and embarrassed to be seen in public, and you'll start to enjoy wearing flattering clothes. Men start to tuck their shirts into their pants, and women find their muumuu days are over. You'll start to feel proud of your body, and you may feel far more comfortable having sex. Life with your partner may be better than ever.

The bad news

After your surgery, you may be so thrilled with your weight loss and all the attention you're suddenly getting that you may find yourself at best distracted and at worst following through with some flirtations you never engaged in before.

After weight loss surgery, both men and women can go a bit crazy as a result of hormone imbalances triggered by rapid weight loss. You may experience super-PMS symptoms, which cause you to lash out at anyone, or you may find yourself feeling very emotional. Guys, this is not just a female thing — expect your emotions to go a bit haywire too. Nothing seems the same — and that's because nothing *is* the same. Even the most patient spouses may begin to wonder if the surgery was worth it!

If you're in a bad marriage before your surgery, don't look to weight loss surgery to save your relationship. In fact, the stress of the surgery will put extra strain on the relationship.

It takes a very secure spouse to feel proud when his or her mate is being openly admired, possibly for the first time. Well-intentioned people may tease your spouse and say, "Hey, your other half looks great. You better watch her!" Those kinds of comments don't help, and they may only add to your spouse's insecurities (or bring them on if they aren't already there).

When your spouse tries to sabotage your experience

In some situations, a spouse may be so opposed to his partner's weight loss surgery that he actually tries to sabotage the patient's efforts to lose weight. If you have a weakness for a certain food, your spouse may intentionally keep that food in the house. Your spouse may suggest going out to eat in restaurants more frequently or express concern about how little you're eating and urge you to eat more. Or your spouse may complain that you don't look good as a thinner person.

There are all kinds of reasons why a spouse may act in such a way. Your spouse may be worried that you'll leave. You may be getting attention from the opposite sex that you never got before, and your spouse may not like it.

If you're having problems with your spouse attempting to sabotage your post-surgery lifestyle, consider the following:

- Are your problems longstanding and just getting worse since your surgery?

- Is your spouse threatening your health by failing to understand the importance of your being at a healthy weight?

- Are you and your spouse willing to consider counseling?

- Are you willing to give up the relationship?

As tragic as it may seem, if your problems are overwhelming, if counseling is not working, leaving your relationship may be the only option.

Weight loss surgery makes good marriages better and bad marriages worse. Unfortunately, the incidence of divorce among weight loss surgery patients is higher than the average. Many times a spouse just can't accept how the relationship has changed because the other spouse has changed so rapidly and completely. Those changes aren't reversible, and the marriage may dissolve.

What you can do to keep your marriage strong

You may be wondering if the future of your marriage is up in the air — all this talk of changes and stresses may make you feel as though you have no say in what happens after your surgery. It's true that you're in your marriage with your spouse, so it isn't *all* within your control, but if you talk openly and honestly with each other about how you're feeling, and if you're committed to making things work, you have a good chance.

Here are some concrete strategies that you can use to keep your relationship healthy through this period of drastic change:

- **Involve your spouse in your plans for surgery.** If your spouse isn't ready for you to have surgery, consider delaying it for a few months until your spouse has a greater level of comfort. In addition to giving your spouse time to get used to the idea, your decision will show your spouse that what he or she thinks matters to you and you want to take his or her feelings into consideration every step of the way.

- **Go together to support-group meetings so your spouse can meet other spouses and hear the positive stories of other patients.** Your spouse may find out about the emotional turmoil you'll be going through after the surgery, which will make him or her better prepared to help you.

- **Reassure your spouse of your love.** Your spouse may be feeling very confused and insecure. When you're going through weight loss surgery, it's very easy to be focused solely on yourself — and for good reason: You're about to undergo a major life change. But keeping your spouse's feelings in mind is important. A hug and an "I love you" go a long way. *Remember:* Just as you need your spouse's support, your spouse needs support from you.

Some people approach surgery hoping that their spouses will love them more or hoping they'll win the approval of their spouses. "If I look better, he'll love me more," or "When I'm thinner, I can be a real man to my wife."

True love or the best you can do?

Many people who are overweight suffer from low self-esteem, and because of this low self-esteem, they may find themselves settling for less-than-ideal or even abusive relationships. As a weight loss surgery patient, you need to think back to how you really felt when you and your spouse first met, fell in love, and got married. Reflect upon what the driving force in the relationship is.

Do some real soul searching and figure out if any of the following applies:

✔ You feel that no one else will love you.

✔ You feel that you don't deserve anything better.

✔ You have a fear of intimacy.

If any of these statements sounds like it describes you, seek out counseling before your surgery. The psychologist who is part of your bariatric team probably has a lot of experience with similar situations, and he's there to help with problems just like this.

You may find that, as you lose weight, you feel much more confident about yourself and you realize that you do deserve much better. *Remember:* To be really successful with weight loss surgery, you want to surround yourself with health — a healthy body, a healthy mind, and healthy relationships.

If you have weight loss surgery, it has to be because it's right for *you,* not because you're hoping to please someone else. If your spouse doesn't love you before the surgery, losing weight won't help — your spouse has to appreciate the wonderful person you are inside, no matter what you weigh.

Parenting and Pregnancy

Children can be a tremendous support after weight loss surgery — they loved you before the surgery and they'll love you after. But even though they may put on brave faces, your kids may have questions, worries, and fears after your surgery, and you need to make sure they feel safe no matter what. In the following sections, we show you how.

We also fill you in on the important topic of pregnancy after weight loss surgery. Prior to your surgery, you may have experienced fertility problems that made getting pregnant difficult. After your surgery, you may have an easier time getting pregnant. But when can you safely start trying? In this section, we give you the information you need if you're thinking about trying to conceive.

Being there for your kids after your surgery

A parent undergoing surgery can be a very frightening experience for children. Your kids may not yet understand the importance of long-term health — so they may not know why you're putting yourself through surgery. They may realize that surgery is risky, and that realization may trigger all kinds of fears.

After your surgery, your kids will definitely notice that you're changing rapidly. You're different from the way you used to be — and your kids may not like that at first. Like adults, children get their security from things staying the same. The changes you go through after surgery may frighten your kids.

You can't expect your kids to understand your decision if you don't take the time to explain it to them. If you're open and honest with them, answering all their questions and giving them the reassurance they need, your kids will adapt to the changes they see.

If you start to feel guilty because of the anxiety your surgery is causing your kids, just remember that, in time, your decision to improve your life with weight loss surgery will be a great lesson for your kids — they may not see it right away, but in time, they'll be proud of you for taking charge of your life.

As you lose weight, your kids may have some behavioral issues. Think about whether you were the parent that your children took after the most. If you and your child were heavy, and you've lost weight, who does your child identify with now? Sometimes both parents have weight loss surgery, but the children are still heavy. Identity issues may arise and have to be dealt with. Tell your kids that you had weight loss surgery for your health, and be sure they know that you aren't rejecting them. Maybe your child was your eating buddy and now you don't eat the way you used to. Make time for your child and do other activities together instead.

Try to stay positive when you tell your children that you're going to have surgery. If surgery is new to your family, emphasize all the good things that'll happen to your family life after. Remind them that

✔ You'll be able to play with them more than you could before surgery.

✔ You'll be able to go on roller coasters and other amusement-park rides with them.

✔ You'll be able to take walks together and ride bikes together.

✔ You'll feel better, and you won't be so grouchy.

Going it alone: Giving your kids what they need when you're a single parent

As a single parent, you may have a really tough time deciding whether to have weight loss surgery. How do the risks of not surviving the surgery stack up against the benefits of a healthier, longer life? If something happens to you, who will raise your children? On the other hand, if you don't have your surgery, and you face increasing health problems, will you be able to be there for your kids?

Here are some things to consider if you're facing weight loss surgery as a single parent:

✔ **Discuss with your surgeon exactly what risks you face.** Most deaths associated with weight loss surgery occur when the health of the patient is very poor going into the surgery. Your surgeon may tell you that if you don't have the surgery, you'll die. If that's the case, your decision has just been made.

✔ **If you decide on surgery, work on conditioning yourself going in.** Even losing 10 or 20 pounds will make for a safer surgery. Do breathing exercises and any conditioning exercises that you can. You can find more on this topic in Chapter 8.

✔ **Delay surgery until your children are a little more independent or you can ensure their future a little more.** If waiting is an option, you may feel better about having the surgery if you wait until your kids are a little older. Talk with your surgeon about the pros and cons of waiting.

✔ **Stay positive.** Your mental health can impact your outcome. When you've decided to go ahead with the surgery, make sure you focus on all the benefits you *and* your kids will see after you've recovered.

Don't be afraid to ask for help. Turn to your local support group — support groups are wonderful sources of information and assistance of all kinds, but they can be a great place to get specific help in addressing your kids' needs. Ask how other parents handled telling their children about surgery and what was especially helpful. Try to find another patient who has a child about the same age as yours, and find out what worked and what didn't.

Your surgeon's practice may have an entire support group devoted to the topic of helping kids cope with a parent's surgery. If your child is a little older, consider taking him or her to a meeting to see and hear from other patients who survived and thrived.

Considering pregnancy after your surgery

"Can I get pregnant?" is one of the most frequently asked questions about weight loss surgery. For some reason, there is a misconception that weight loss surgery and pregnancy are mutually exclusive, when just the opposite is true. Weight loss surgery involves surgery on the abdominal area and small intestines, which, in terms of anatomy, are far away from the uterus.

Women who have weight loss surgery and reach a normal weight go on to have very healthy and normal pregnancies. They have lower-risk pregnancies because they're carrying less weight; their blood pressure is lower; they're on fewer medications; their health in general is better; and they find it easier to exercise throughout their pregnancies.

That said, the timing of a pregnancy is very critical following surgery. Many women going into weight loss surgery have long believed that they're infertile because they haven't been able to conceive for so long and have become accustomed to unprotected sex. After weight loss surgery, however, many women find that they have newfound or increased fertility and can become pregnant when they've never been able to conceive in the past.

Added to this new fertility is the fact that, as you lose weight, you like yourself better, you feel healthier, and you naturally feel sexier. Chances are, you're having more sex. If it's unprotected sex, your chances of becoming pregnant are greater than they were before surgery.

We recommend avoiding pregnancy during the first year after your surgery, while you're still losing weight. In fact, to be on the safe side, wait 12 to 18 months. During that time, you're eating only enough to sustain yourself — you aren't eating enough to nurture a growing fetus. The chief concern following gastric bypass or duodenal switch surgeries is deficiencies in vitamin B12 and folic acid, so if you decide to get pregnant, be sure to take extra supplements — talk to your surgeon and obstetrician about your unique needs.

The first year after surgery is also when losing weight will be the easiest and fastest. Because it will never be this easy again, you want to take advantage of that time and lose as much weight as you possibly can. When you've reached a healthier weight, you'll be in the best shape possible to care for your infant.

As always, talk with your doctors about when you can safely start to try to get pregnant. And be sure that your obstetrician knows that you've had weight loss surgery. Your obstetrician and your surgeon will want to consult so that you'll have the safest pregnancy possible.

If you have persistent vague abdominal complaints, let both your surgeon and obstetrician know. You can get lab tests and ultrasounds to check out how you are. X-rays are usually discouraged during pregnancy, but sometimes they're necessary to best identify the problem.

The Dating Game: Taking Yourself off the Bench

As you start to lose weight, you may notice something: People are noticing *you* — but this time, it's in a *good* way. You no longer have that feeling that people are staring, laughing to themselves, and thinking, "What's wrong with her?" or "Doesn't he have any control?" Instead, you have the suspicion that they're looking and thinking, "Hey, she looks pretty good" or "Wow, what a hunk." You've lost weight, you carry yourself differently, and your confidence has increased — and confidence can be very attractive. You may have the offer of dates for the first time *ever*.

Dating can be fun, but it also can be an emotional challenge. If you're single, issues of intimacy can be very scary. You may have lost a lot of weight and look terrific with clothes on, but take those clothes off and your confidence sags along with those folds of skin. Just facing that prospect can keep you at home alone in front of the TV on a Saturday night.

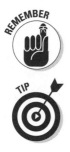

Nobody's body is perfect, but for the weight loss surgery patient with low self-esteem and a poor sense of body image, those perceptions of imperfection can be exaggerated. The pounds are gone, but you haven't been touched by a plastic surgeon, and that loose skin isn't pretty. That's the time to appreciate what an accomplishment it is to have lost so much weight.

If it's been a long time since you last dated, or if you've never dated before, here are some tips to consider as you approach dating:

- **Take your time.** Don't rush into a relationship thinking your first relationship will be your best and last. You may have settled for anything you could get in the past. Be sure this relationship is what you really want before you start planning the wedding.

- **Think about how much you want to share.** How much and how soon will you tell your date about your surgery? Some patients are very proud of losing so much weight. Others are embarrassed that they were "failures" for such a long time. Think ahead of time about how you'll handle that issue — and remember that there is no right way: Just do what feels best to you.

- **If you're going to keep your surgery private, don't go out to eat on your first date.** You'll be nibbling, and your date will definitely notice. What could be worse is if you talk and eat at the same time and find it necessary to run to the bathroom because you've gotten something stuck. Instead, consider dates that are built around other activities — like going for a walk or a bike ride, or taking in a movie or a concert.

✔ **Before you start dating, think about what you'll use to cope if the relationship goes wrong.** You can't use food anymore. Put some thought into that just to be on the safe side. We're not saying you should go into a first date assuming you won't have a good time or even start a relationship — keep a positive, but realistic attitude. Know that, just as with your weight loss surgery journey, the journey of dating has its ups and downs and anticipating them is half the battle.

The whole issue of dating is a complex one. For more information on this intriguing and sometimes scary subject, we recommend *Dating For Dummies*, 3rd Edition, by Joy Browne, PhD (Wiley).

That's What Friends Are For

Groups of friends are often the same size with the same interests. As you start to think about having weight loss surgery, and if you're the first person in your group to consider it, you may be met with a lot of resistance from other members of the group.

Take a look at where the resistance is coming from. Are you the largest person in your circle of friends? If so, after the surgery you'll no longer have that distinction — someone else will be the largest person in the group, and you can bet that person won't like it.

Just as you may find some friends who are less than supportive with your decision to have weight loss surgery, other friends will be behind you 100 percent — and you'll wonder how you ever could have gotten through the surgery without them.

In the following sections, we give you some tips for telling your friends about your surgery and working through the effects your surgery may have on your friendships.

Sharing your decision with your friends

How you tell your friends about your decision to have weight loss surgery can have a huge effect on whether you keep those friends. If you try the following strategies, things may go more smoothly:

✔ **Explain to your friends how you came to the decision to have surgery.**

✔ **Share your current health concerns and advice that your physician has given to you.**

✔ **Invite your friends along to a support-group meeting.** If one of your friends is especially close to you, arrange for him or her to go with you on an appointment with your surgeon.

✔ **Share this book with your friends so they're as well informed as you are.** The more knowledge they have, the more supportive they'll be.

✔ **Ask your support-group leader to devote a meeting to this topic, and see if any other patients would consider having an informal meeting to talk about the issue.**

✔ **If your friendships seem strained, ask your friends if they'll consider going with you to a counseling session with the staff counselor in the bariatric practice.** Friends can be as important in your life as family, and doing everything you can to save your friendships may be important.

Knowing what may change after your surgery

What do friends often do together? They go out to eat. After surgery, your capacity to eat is greatly diminished for at least the first year. When your friends invite you out following your surgery and all you can eat is a portion of an appetizer while they're devouring a super-supreme pizza, they may feel uncomfortable. Plus, after your surgery, going out to eat just won't have the allure that it used to, especially for the first few months.

Weight loss surgery patients find that they have renewed energy and want to try some activities that they haven't been able to do in years. Instead of going out to eat with your friends, you may want to go bike riding or hiking, or just do something physically challenging.

Help your friends understand that they're still important in your life. Yes, you've changed, but inside you're still the same. Talk with them frankly about how important this new way of living is to you and, with any luck, they'll love you enough to give you the space to explore your new interests. Who knows? They may follow in your footsteps — but just remember it has to be in their own time.

All in the Extended Family: Dealing with the Archie Bunkers in Your World

Extended family members can be your biggest fans and supporters as you go through your surgical journey — or they can be a real challenge to deal with. Family dynamics may exist that have nothing to do with you, but that you somehow find yourself in the middle of.

In families, everyone seems to have a specific role to play. When you step out of that role and make a big change, other family members will notice, and you may not receive all the positive support you need and want.

Fending off attacks

Genetics plays a role in obesity, which means you probably have many relatives who are in need of weight loss surgery. Those relatives may feel the need to justify themselves and their decision not to have the surgery by expressing negative comments to or about you. Although these comments can hurt, sometimes it helps if you try to figure out why they haven't had weight loss surgery themselves:

- They may be uninformed and believe that weight loss surgery today is as ineffective and dangerous as it was 20 years ago.
- They may be in denial about their own weight.
- They may not have the courage to make such a life-altering change.
- They may be happy with their weight.

Regardless of why they've opted not to have the surgery themselves, they may resent you for going ahead with it yourself. **Remember:** The remarks they make are less about you and more about how they feel about themselves.

In dealing with extended family members (whether they're overweight themselves or not), arm yourself with knowledge and be willing to discuss any of their objections. As they see you succeed with your weight loss, become much healthier, and then maintain that weight loss, they'll be proud of you — as they should be.

Notice something different? What to do when they don't even notice

Instead of having to deal with family members who attack your decision to have the surgery, you may be faced with family members who don't seem to notice that you're losing weight. You may be having terrific success and find that your family doesn't say a word. First, you may wonder if maybe you don't look as good as you think you do. But then, after a while, you realize that the family members are just choosing to stay mute on the subject.

Ignoring your success can be just as hurtful as attacking your decision. Silence can mean one of several things:

- ✔ They're trying to be polite and not talk about your weight.
- ✔ They've seen you lose weight and regain it and are just expecting you to go back to your former size.
- ✔ They're so envious that they just can't speak.
- ✔ They truly haven't noticed.

Depending on your relationship with your family members, you can decide either to ignore their reaction (or lack thereof) or to talk to them about it. If their lack of response is really bothering you, try bringing up the subject. You might say, "Hey, did you know I've lost X pounds?" If they just didn't notice or they were trying to be polite by not talking about it, you can bet they'll let their enthusiasm show. If they're envious of you or otherwise upset, they may not react very well — but you can always use that as an opportunity to get things out in the open. Try saying, "Something seems to be bothering you. Can we talk about that?"

You can't force your family members to react the way you want them to. And if some of them aren't as supportive as you hoped they'd be, try to focus your time and attention on those who *do* give you the support you need. Your other family members may come around in time.

Chapter 22

Now That I'm Thin, What about the Skin?

Your skin is the largest organ in your body, and after working hard to lose so much weight, you may be discouraged to find that your skin drapes down in unattractive folds or looks damaged with stretch marks. This doesn't happen to everyone, but if it happens to you, what do you do about it? Do you live with it or do you have it taken care of through plastic surgery?

Excess skin isn't just a cosmetic issue. If your skin starts to sag, hygiene can become a major problem. Any skin fold can be prone to rashes, which are usually a type of yeast infection. Common areas are under the breasts, in the belly button, and above the pubic area and groin. Yeast infections occur because these areas get very hot and moist. Using an antifungal powder and keeping the area dry can help, but if the problem is something you battle continuously, you may decide to opt for surgery.

Chafing is another major problem. It can occur between the thighs, under the arms, and in areas that rub against the bra. Wearing longer, fitted garments on the arms and legs can decrease irritation and breakdown of the skin in these areas, but again, you may decide that surgery is your best option.

Plastic surgery following weight loss surgery often requires individualized body contouring. In body contouring, excess skin and pockets of fat are removed from the abdominal area, thighs, buttocks, upper arms, and breasts. It's a total reworking of the body, and it's becoming more popular. That said, body contouring can require several days of hospitalization, six weeks off work, and a year for the scars to heal. A complete body contouring with a face lift can cost at least $30,000. The total number of surgeries is usually spread over several months.

The plastic surgery procedure will most likely be more painful than your weight loss surgery.

In this chapter, we let you know what you can expect, your surgical options, how to find a plastic surgeon, and what kind of results you can anticipate.

Knowing Whether You'll Need Plastic Surgery

It would be nice if your skin just snapped back to where it should be, but that doesn't always happen. Your skin is like a balloon that you blow up and deflate. When you lose a huge amount of weight, your skin can look like that deflated balloon.

The good news is that not everyone who has weight loss surgery will require plastic surgery. Before you lose all your weight, you can't really be sure whether you'll need it. Although there are no guarantees, here are some factors that affect whether you'll need plastic surgery:

- ✔ **Your age:** People who are younger have more elasticity in their skin, and their skin snaps back more easily.

- ✔ **How much weight you have to lose:** The more overweight you are, the more your skin is stretched, and the more likely you are to need plastic surgery.

- ✔ **How many times you've gained and lost weight in your lifetime:** Your skin is like that balloon that goes up and down. The stretching and deflating cause the skin to lose elasticity.

- ✔ **Where you carry your weight:** If the majority of your weight is concentrated in one area, such as your abdominal area, rather than all over your body, then your chances of needing plastic surgery are increased.

- ✔ **Whether you've ever smoked:** Smoking breaks down *collagen,* a major component of skin and other structural components of the body. Smokers develop more loose skin than nonsmokers do.

- ✔ **Whether your skin has been exposed to a lot of sun over the years:** All that lying out in the sun makes your skin less elastic.

- ✔ **Your skin type:** Some skin types have more elasticity than others. Genetics plays a part.

Looking at Steps You Can Take

It would be nice if there were something you could do about hanging skin, short of plastic surgery, but generally there is not. Although exercise will help your weight loss, it won't do anything for your excess skin. What exercise *can* do is give you very nice, well-defined muscles under all that skin, which can help fill out the sag. There are some newer ultrasound technologies to reduce skin sag without any cutting of your skin, but check with a plastic surgeon to see if this could help you.

Hydration and the elasticity of your skin go hand in hand. Be sure that your skin stays well hydrated by drinking lots of water.

In the months leading up to plastic surgery, doing the following will help give you better results:

- ✔ Exercise so your muscles are toned.

- ✔ Eat a lot of protein so you'll heal faster.

- ✔ Be as close to your goal weight as possible.

- ✔ Take all your vitamins so you're healthy.

- ✔ Don't smoke. Smoking will directly affect your ability to heal. As you smoke, less oxygen is available for the healing process, and removing pounds of skin requires a lot of healing.

As you lose weight, before you have plastic surgery, you may find that your hanging skin significantly impacts what clothes you can wear, and your clothing size can vary because of the "spare tire" you're carrying. You can find many different elastic or spandex girdles to strap yourself in and give yourself a smoother silhouette — and these can really be effective. Some new options are available for guys, too, including ones from SPANX (go to www.spanx.com and click the SPANX for Men link).

Knowing How Long to Wait before Plastic Surgery

In general, you should wait to have plastic surgery until your weight has been stable (meaning, you've stopped losing weight, and it's at the level it's going to be) for at least three to six months. You don't want to have plastic surgery too soon, because if you lose additional weight, your skin will start to sag again.

You may have trouble knowing whether you're at your lowest weight or whether you've just hit a very stubborn plateau. If you aren't at your goal weight, keep trying to lose more weight. Don't give up on yourself too easily.

In addition to waiting until your weight has been stable for three to six months, you need to give your body a chance to heal from the weight loss surgery. You want to be in very good physical shape going into plastic surgery. You need to be eating enough nutrients in order for healing to take place.

The bottom line: You want to wait until your weight has stabilized and your obesity-related health problems have improved or been cured. The more physically fit you are, the healthier you are and the better your chances for success.

Choosing a Plastic Surgeon

Plastic surgery for weight loss surgery patients is a very specific subspecialty of plastic surgery. But you have options and special considerations when it comes to who will do your plastic surgery.

You may want your bariatric surgeon to perform your plastic surgery. For example, if you have a lot of hanging skin in your abdominal area even before you start to lose weight, some surgeons will remove that excess skin at the same time as your weight loss surgery. This doesn't happen often, but it is a possibility, and your general health is definitely a factor. Your surgeon will not do this if it puts you at risk. *Remember:* After you lose all your weight, you may need additional plastic surgery.

You also may want to have your bariatric surgeon do plastic surgery for you if you develop a hernia after your weight loss surgery and need additional surgery to have the hernia repaired. The bariatric surgeon may be able to do plastic surgery while operating to repair the hernia.

Although you may be most comfortable sticking with your bariatric surgeon for plastic surgery, keep in mind that your bariatric surgeon is not a plastic surgeon, so the results will not be perfect.

Also, keep in mind that, if your insurance company won't cover your plastic surgery, and you have it done during another procedure (for example, the repair of a hernia), you'll still have to pay for the plastic-surgery portion of the operation and the related portion of the anesthesia, operating room, and hospital stay.

For the best results, you should have your surgery performed by a plastic surgeon who has experience working with weight loss surgery patients. The work that you'll need to have done is very different from cosmetic nip-and-tuck surgery and also very different from reconstructive surgery done as a result of accidents or birth defects.

Here are ways to find a good plastic surgeon:

- ✔ **Ask your bariatric surgeon for a referral.** Your bariatric surgeon will probably have a professional relationship with experts in the field.

- ✔ **Ask for referrals at your support group.** Someone in the support group most likely has had plastic surgery. Ask for recommendations, and find out about the results.

- ✔ **Attend support-group meetings when plastic surgeons make presentations there.** You'll have an opportunity to see slides of their work, ask questions, and get a feel for how you like the surgeon. Just one more reason to join a support group!

- ✔ **Contact the American Society of Plastic Surgeons.** This professional association operates a website at www.plasticsurgery.org, where you can find board-certified plastic surgeons in your geographic area. When speaking to the plastic surgeon, be sure to ask what his or her experience with weight loss surgery patients is. Ask for references from patients who have had weight loss surgery. *Remember:* Because of privacy laws, the surgeon may not be able to give you references unless patients have volunteered to be contacted.

When you meet with your plastic surgeon, be prepared to be photographed in very little clothing. Although you may feel very embarrassed, the surgeon uses these photos to additionally plan the surgery, for documentation for insurance purposes, and for a comparison after the surgery.

Be sure your surgeon understands that he may not use your photographs on the Internet or in any promotion without your written approval. Then be careful what you sign.

Figuring Out How You'll Pay for Plastic Surgery

Insurance companies apply the rule of "medical necessity" when considering whether they'll pay for plastic surgery. They will never cover plastic surgery if they consider it cosmetic. They often will provide coverage if it's reconstructive surgery.

The American Medical Association in 1989 adopted the following definitions:

- *Cosmetic surgery* is performed to reshape structures of the body in order to improve the patient's appearance and self-esteem.

- *Reconstructive surgery* is performed on abnormal structures of the body, caused by congenital defect, developmental abnormality, trauma, infection, tumor, or disease. It's generally performed to improve function, but it may also be done to approximate a normal appearance.

Here are some arguments for insurance coverage:

- You have rashes that won't heal as a result of excess skin.

- You get frequent yeast infections because of excess skin.

- You've tried treatments for these problems that haven't worked.

- You have *skin breakdown,* where the skin is worn away from rubbing.

- Your skin inhibits your ability to walk, to work, or to have a normal life.

- You have hygiene problems because of excess skin.

- Your breasts or your *pannus* (the large flap of hanging skin of the abdomen that sometimes forms after massive weight loss) are so heavy that you're having severe back problems.

Getting plastic surgery covered by insurance is never easy. All your problems will have to be well documented by your doctor. Some plans are more lenient than others. You may have to work hard justifying your reasons with your insurance company.

Even if you have to pay for your plastic surgery out of your own pocket, check with your accountant. The cost may be tax deductible if it's used to correct a problem related to obesity. If it's a purely cosmetic procedure, you're out of luck.

Looking At the Different Plastic Surgery Procedures

Many patients want all their plastic surgery done at once. They want to get it all over with for a variety of reasons. Splitting up the surgery is more expensive — you have more hospital time and more anesthesia time. If you split up your surgery, you also have the inconvenience of having to recuperate twice.

Following the advice of your plastic surgeon is important. If the surgery can be done all at once, your surgeon will let you know. If the advice is to do the work in two separate procedures, don't push for one. During plastic surgery, you have a lot of fluid changes and you can lose a fair amount of blood. If you lose too much blood, it can be dangerous. *Remember:* A good plastic surgeon is most concerned about your health and safety; if your surgeon recommends splitting up the surgeries, do what she recommends.

Although plastic surgeons can give you incredible results, discuss your expectations with your surgeon. You'll have scarring and you likely won't have the body of someone who is half your age. All the years of an unhealthy lifestyle or the inability to exercise regularly may have taken its toll on your body. Your body won't be perfect, but it will be much different following your surgery.

As with any surgery, things can go wrong. Here are some problems to prepare for:

✔ **You may have a *seroma* (a collection of fluid under the skin that is not drained by tubes).** Seromas are drained with a small needle in your surgeon's office. They aren't serious, but they do need to be followed by your surgeon.

✔ **Infection is possible, because you'll have extensive incisions.** Any open wound is vulnerable to infection, and plastic surgery is no different.

✔ **When the skin is pulled very tight, there is the possibility of the incision opening or part of the skin dying.** When this happens, the healing time is very slow — but you will heal.

✔ **You may have numbness, which can be a problem in any plastic surgery.** Nerve endings are cut during the surgery and, although the feeling normally returns, sometimes it doesn't.

✔ **You may experience excessive bleeding or blood clots in the legs.** Both of these problems will need prompt attention from your surgeon.

In the following sections, we cover some plastic surgery procedures common among weight loss surgery patients.

Panniculectomy and abdominoplasty: Losing your gut

The most common area of hanging skin is in the abdominal area. The flap of skin, or apron, that hangs down over this area is called a *pannus*. In some people, the flap of skin hangs down only a few inches; in others, it hangs well into the thigh area. Excess skin here can be very troublesome, often interfering with walking. This area is also prone to yeast infections and rashes, often to the point that corrective surgery is considered a medical necessity by insurance companies. The surgery to remove this excess skin is technically called a *panniculectomy*.

An *abdominoplasty* is more extensive and involves tightening the muscles of the abdomen. The incision is normally horizontal, which is easier to hide, but if you have a lot of skin to remove, the incision may have a vertical component. You also may lose your belly button in the process. Although the belly button serves no purpose, some people feel odd not having one. Don't worry — the plastic surgeon can make you another one if you want.

Following surgery, you may be required to wear a tight binder. The binder helps to ease swelling, helps with the pain, and provides support to your tissues while they're healing.

These surgeries generally take two to eight hours and require an overnight stay in the hospital. After surgery, you'll likely be sent home with two drainage tubes, which remove the excess fluid and need to be emptied twice a day. You'll need the tubes for about a week, or until there is little fluid to drain.

Breast reconstruction

The surgeries available are a breast lift and a breast reduction, which are entirely different surgeries:

- ✔ **Breast lift:** A *breast lift* is designed to pull the breasts up so they don't sag so much. This procedure is cosmetic, which means your insurance company likely won't cover it.

- ✔ **Breast reduction:** A *breast reduction* is a surgery to reduce the size of your breasts. Large breasts are heavy and can cause upper-back pain. This surgery may be covered by insurance. In order for the procedure to be approved by your insurance company, you have to show infections in the folds under the breasts, back pain related to the weight of the breasts, or grooves in the shoulder region related to bra straps.

Brachioplasty: Removing those nasty bat wings

Weight loss surgery patients often are bothered by excess skin that hangs down from the upper arm, often referred to as "bat wings." The surgery that removes that excess skin is known as *brachioplasty*.

The scar in this surgery is difficult to hide, because it runs the length of the inside of the upper arm. In some cases, the surgeon is able to hide the scar in the armpit.

Lower-body lift

Your thighs and buttocks can end up looking pretty sad following surgery, as all the skin responds to gravity. The thighs can be an additional source of rash and infection, because walking causes lots of rubbing.

The procedure to correct these areas combined with the abdomen is known as a *lower-body lift*. The thighs and butt are corrected by pulling up the skin very tightly, somewhat like putting on a pair of pants, and cutting off the excess.

Face lifts and neck lifts

Some patients opt to have work done on their faces and necks because excessive weight loss has made them look very old. Procedures can include a face lift, brow lift, eye lift, or nose job (technically called a *rhinoplasty*). The muscles and the skin are stretched to smooth out the skin and make it tight. For the face lift, the incision is made just in front of the ear, and any scarring occurs behind the ear. For the brow lift, the scar is in the hairline.

Following a face lift or similar procedure, you can expect to have considerable swelling and bruising. (You can use stage makeup to hide some of the bruising.) You'll have black eyes and a swollen, bruised face for a couple weeks. Warn your family that they'll be suspected of abuse.

Liposuction

Liposuction is a procedure in which the surgeon sucks out fat from under your skin with a long tube. Liposuction is used in combination with other procedures for weight loss surgery patients and not as a procedure by itself. Liposuction does not help sagging skin. It's used to smooth out your skin followed by removing and stretching the excess skin.

Considering Botox and fillers

After significant weight loss, patients sometimes describe their skin as being deflated. Wrinkles appear where they didn't have them before or become more prominent. Botox and fillers can help.

Botox is a medication that can be used to decrease the number of wrinkles on your face. Botox is injected into different muscle groups like the ones that give your forehead wrinkles, frown lines, and those small wrinkles around the eyes known as crow's feet. Doesn't sound pretty, does it? The medication acts to stop the muscles from flexing, which can cause the wrinkles. It usually lasts for three to four months and is helpful for some weight loss surgery patients.

Fillers are collagen-based products that can be used to fill in the lines on your face, including smile lines or those deep furrows in your brow. These products are expensive and last approximately nine months.

Although Botox and fillers are expensive, using them often helps ward off that face lift and can help with your appearance.

Note: These procedures are considered cosmetic and will not be covered by your insurance.

Knowing What Your Recovery Will Be Like

Most surgeries require approximately four weeks of recovery time. During that time, you're very limited in the weight that you're allowed to lift. The amount of pain involved depends on the type of procedure you have, as well as your own tolerance of pain (or pain threshold). Many patients report that the procedures are very painful — more so than weight loss surgery (especially if the weight loss surgery was performed laparoscopically). Although moving around right away is important, standing up straight may be too painful. Patients tend to go back to work after four to six weeks for most surgeries.

Healing takes time. You may think that you'll look better faster than you really do. You'll have a lot of puffiness that may take two or three months to work out of your system. So, it'll be a while until you see really good results from your plastic surgery.

Any kind of change takes adjustment, even if it's change for the better. Change with plastic surgery is particularly difficult for a couple reasons:

✔ **Everything gets worse before it gets better.** Following plastic surgery, you'll have pain and swelling. You may have drainage tubes and bruising. You may not like the look of the incisions and be concerned about scarring. You may even weigh more than you did before the skin was removed! If you had high hopes of looking good immediately after the surgery, you'll be disappointed and headed for depression.

Give yourself time to heal. Be patient with the process and with yourself. Any extra weight is just from tissue swelling and will come down as you heal.

✔ **Plastic surgery changes your self-image.** Your self-image is fundamental to how you feel about yourself. Even though you look better, you look vastly different. You may feel for a while that you're in someone else's body. If you're bothered by this, talk to your surgeon about getting psychological support (through a counselor and/or support group) as you adjust.

I'm looking at the girl in the mirror . . .

I came from working in the high-end worlds of fashion and magazine publishing and had worked with women for years on better body image as an editor and styling expert. But we all have struggles, and mine was my weight.

In 2000, I hit my highest weight, 289 pounds. In 2008, after eight years of trying to lose weight, I decided to have gastric banding. I'm thankful for the tools and skills I now have after my weight loss surgery, but even having reached a lower weight of 180 pounds, my weight loss journey continues to be a long-term project.

After my weight loss, I was very frustrated with the excess skin that remained on my abdomen and lower hip area, the dermatological skin infections under the hanging belly fat, continuing lower back pain, and really serious pressure on my already compromised bladder.

Weight loss surgery wasn't a magic pill. I still had this upsetting, unpleasant reminder of "what once was." It felt like I would never make peace with the woman in the mirror and that was always my goal. So, I opted for plastic surgery.

With my reconstructive plastic surgeon's help, I was able to rid myself of the last vestiges from decades of being unhealthy, uneasy, and struggling with my weight. Today I have a healthier outlook, and I'm even more confident in my own skin.

Michele Weston
New York, New York

Part VI
The Part of Tens

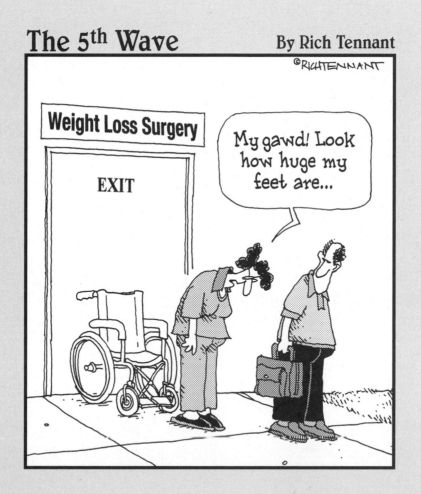

The 5th Wave   By Rich Tennant

Weight Loss Surgery

EXIT

My gawd! Look how huge my feet are...

In this part . . .

No *For Dummies* book is complete without a Part of Tens. Here you'll discover all the misconceptions that people have about weight loss surgery. We also explore all the benefits to your health and overall happiness. But happiness can be short-lived if you don't maintain that weight loss, so we give you tips on how to be successful for the rest of your life.

Chapter 23

Ten Weight Loss Surgery Myths

*W*eight loss surgery is in the news almost daily. You may hear everything from glowing reports of saved lives to horror stories about surgeries gone wrong. No doubt, you know people who have had the surgery or you know someone who knows someone who has had the surgery. And like the game of gossip, reports get distorted. Here are some myths about weight loss surgery that you may have heard — and that we're here to dispel.

You'll Never Regain Your Weight

Weight loss surgery is only a tool — the amount of weight you lose and how much of that weight loss you maintain is up to you. Most patients do regain some weight — some as much as 20 percent to 30 percent, and others even more than that. When you go through weight loss surgery, you have no guarantees that you'll be thin your entire life. But if you eat a healthy diet and follow a good exercise routine, your chances of not regaining weight are greatly improved.

You'll Never Be Hungry

After your weight loss surgery, you *will* experience hunger — but not right away. Soon after surgery, many patients experience what is described as *head hunger,* which is like withdrawal symptoms from food. After your body adjusts to eating such small amounts, you'll feel only very mild sensations of hunger for many months.

A year or two or more after your surgery, you'll definitely experience hunger. But unlike before your surgery, you'll need only a small meal to satisfy that hunger. You'll definitely be able to eat more at one sitting than you could eat right after your surgery — but try to eat for only 20 minutes and limit your snacks. Watching your carbohydrate intake also can help control those hunger pangs.

Weight Loss Surgery Is the Easy Way Out

Nothing angers a weight loss surgery patient more than hearing someone say that weight loss surgery is the easy way out. There is nothing easy about it. Consider the following:

- ✔ You have to go through rigorous physical and psychological testing to ensure that you're an appropriate candidate for surgery.

- ✔ You may have to fight with your insurance company to get the surgery covered.

- ✔ You may face complications from the surgery.

- ✔ You have to endure about four weeks of liquids and pureed foods — not fun!

- ✔ You have to learn a whole new way of eating — and there are consequences if you don't follow the rules. You may throw up, suffer dumping syndrome (see Chapter 18); experience nausea; or get food stuck in your *stoma* (the opening from your new small pouch to your small intestine), above the band, or in your new narrow stomach — and that hurts!

- ✔ As your system adjusts to the surgery, you may have a real problem with nausea.

- ✔ You may lose a lot of your hair for a three- to five-month period after the surgery.

- ✔ When you realize that you can no longer use food for comfort, you have to adjust psychologically and find new ways to cope.

Next time people tell you that weight loss surgery is easy, try naming just a couple items on this list. That'll show 'em — and besides, you'll be educating them so they don't make that comment to someone else in the future.

You Can't Get Pregnant after Weight Loss Surgery

Many patients have trouble getting pregnant prior to surgery and find that they're very fertile following surgery. This is good news if you want to have children — or it may be bad news if you don't.

Contrary to popular belief, pregnancy following weight loss surgery is very possible. Patients are much less at risk during pregnancy because their other health problems have lessened or disappeared. After your weight is back to normal, and assuming you don't have any other health problems, you can expect to have a normal delivery.

If you're a woman of childbearing age, use two forms of birth control for one year following surgery. During that first year, you aren't eating enough to nourish yourself plus a growing fetus, so you don't want to get pregnant then. Besides, you want to concentrate on your own weight loss during that first year. Better safe than sorry.

You'll Be Happy after Surgery

Unhappy people come in all shapes and sizes. Losing weight does not guarantee happiness. That said, you'll find many rewards — both physical and emotional — when you reach a normal weight. You'll have a stronger sense of self-esteem, and your health problems will be much more under control. But weight loss surgery won't solve all your problems, and you don't want to go into it thinking it will.

Weight Loss Surgery Is Very Risky

Many people associate weight loss surgery with a very high risk of death, but that just isn't the reality. The death rate associated with weight loss surgery is considered less than one-third of 1 percent, when the surgery is performed by an experienced surgeon.

Be sure that your surgery is done by an experienced surgeon. Check that your surgeon or the hospital is part of a Center of Excellence. Many studies have shown that surgeons have a learning curve with weight loss surgery. The more surgeries a surgeon has performed, the safer you're likely to be. (For more on choosing a surgeon, turn to Chapter 5.)

Also, consider the health risks of staying severely obese. You may be at far greater risk staying that way than you will be having surgery.

You'll Have a Great Body

Following weight loss surgery, you'll lose a lot of weight in the form of fat, but you won't necessarily have a great-looking body. As you lose weight, your skin won't necessarily shrink along with your body, which may leave you with lots of sagging skin. Exercise will tone your muscles and help you lose even more weight, but it will do nothing for your skin. You may need to resort to having plastic surgery to deal with excess skin — this just depends on your own body and how it responds after surgery.

You may not have the perfect body, but you'll be healthy!

You Can't Eat for the Rest of Your Life

You can eat very normally after weight loss surgery; in fact, many patients say that they enjoy eating *more* after the surgery than they did before. They're able to savor their food because they aren't so concerned about consuming huge amounts.

True, in the first few months, you aren't enjoying eating. But after your first year, you'll be able to eat almost anything, just in smaller amounts.

Weight Loss Surgery Will Save Your Marriage

Actually, the opposite is true. The divorce rate among couples in which one has had weight loss surgery is higher than the average. Many couples aren't able to weather the drastic change that happens when one spouse loses a tremendous amount of weight. Your spouse may become jealous of the new attention that you're receiving. Or you may find that with improved self-esteem, you're no longer willing to endure treatment that you don't find acceptable. Or, with a whole new appearance, your personality may change — and your spouse may not like that new personality.

Be ready to seek out counseling if it looks like your marriage is headed for trouble. Try to involve your spouse as much as possible by talking about the ways that you're changing. Although the surgery won't save a marriage, it can make good marriages even better.

You Have to Pay for Weight Loss Surgery Yourself

You *may* have to pay for your own weight loss surgery, but weight loss surgery often is covered by insurance. Even though, in recent years, insurance companies have become more demanding in their screening of patients, the vast majority of surgeries are covered.

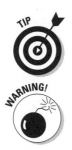 If any of your co-workers has had weight loss surgery, ask about his or her experience with insurance coverage. You'll get a sense of what, if anything, you may be up against.

If you have the same insurance company as one of your friends but you aren't on the same plan, your insurance could be entirely different. One employer may list the surgery as an exclusion for its employees, while another employer that uses the same insurance company may not. Just be sure to talk with your insurance company beforehand so you know what costs, if any, will be involved.

Chapter 24

Ten Benefits of Weight Loss Surgery

Weight loss surgery can help you look better and, more important, feel healthier. Successful weight loss surgery patients feel improvements medically, physically, emotionally, and mentally. Countless individuals can relate to one post-op patient's declaration, "Today I am living the life I always dreamed about." In this chapter, we let you know some of the many benefits weight loss surgery may bring.

Effective and Maintained Weight Loss

After years of failing to lose weight with yo-yo dieting, commercial weight-loss programs, fads, and exercise, you have a newfound hope when you choose to have weight loss surgery. Studies have shown that the majority of severely obese people who lose weight without having surgery regain most the weight lost over the next five years. Sound familiar?

Weight loss typically occurs quickly after obesity surgery and usually continues for one and a half to two years. Weight loss surgery is currently the only treatment available that has been found to be effective as a long-term treatment for severe obesity.

Improved Quality and Quantity of Life

You'll feel better physically and emotionally when your weight is under control. Many people report having developed a newfound sense of well-being after surgery. You may discover outside interests as your focus on food diminishes. As you lose significant amounts of weight, you'll have more energy. The shortness of breath associated with everyday activities — such as walking, playing with children, or doing housework — disappears. You experience and enjoy an amazing freedom from living a lifestyle where food is an afterthought, not the driving force. Many people find improvement in their professional and social lives, too. And studies show that patients live longer than those whose severe obesity is left untreated.

Better Appetite Control

Most people who've had weight loss surgery find that they don't experience the hunger they had prior to surgery. They start to become less preoccupied with food. This decrease in hunger helps you stick to your new eating plan, as well as your exercise and behavior modifications. The focus is on your health, not on hunger.

Improved Obesity-Related Health Issues

Your obesity-related health problems will likely improve and/or be easier to control with fewer medications if you lose weight. You can expect to experience a remission or improvement in the following conditions:

- High blood pressure
- Joint and back pain associated with obesity
- Diabetes
- Sleep apnea
- High cholesterol
- Heart disease
- Symptoms of gastroesophageal reflux disease (GERD)
- Respiratory problems
- Osteoarthritis
- Cardiovascular function
- Infertility

TECHNICAL STUFF

We're in the money: Economic benefits

According to the American Society for Metabolic & Bariatric Surgery (ASMBS), prescription-drug expenditures account for greater than 15 percent of annual healthcare spending and account for nearly 10 percent of total healthcare expenditures in the United States. With successful weight loss surgery, your medical problems will typically improve or go away — and quickly. Prescription costs are directly related to obesity and the problems associated with obesity.

Weight loss surgery often prevents patients from requiring expensive operations for other medical problems. Many obese people experience joint-related problems with their knees, hips, or backs. Many orthopedic surgeons are hesitant to operate on someone's back or knee unless the patient has been able to lose weight. With weight loss surgery, you're less likely to require joint-related surgery. But if you do need joint-related surgery, your recovery will be improved after you've lost weight.

Plus, living as a thin person costs less. In addition to reductions in grocery bills, you'll be avoiding hundreds and sometimes thousands of dollars per year in prescription medications, doctor's visits, and obesity-related medical costs. (See the nearby sidebar, "We're in the money: Economic benefits," for more information.)

Improved Self-Esteem

Feelings of guilt, inadequacy, embarrassment, and failure often build up after years of trying and not succeeding at losing weight. With progressive weight loss, you begin to feel proud of the new shape you're attaining. Feelings of self-consciousness and shame are gradually replaced with feelings of confidence and self-control.

Looking Good

Weight loss surgery is more than just losing weight. When you start to lose those pounds, you can't help but feel good about looking slimmer and healthier.

Better Sex

In addition to improvements in self-esteem, mobility, and overall energy, many patients report an increase in their sex drive after weight loss surgery.

Shopping for Regular-Size Clothes

Before surgery, going to the mall and trying to find something that would fit may have been a dreadful experience. No more squeezing into something or buying the biggest size the store offered. Now you have the joy of selecting any item off the rack without fear of it not fitting or being too tight. You may even have the pleasure of saying, "Do you have this in a *smaller* size?"

More Opportunities

Discrimination against the obese is still common. No naturally thin person could ever understand how hard it is to participate in life as a severely obese person. Because of this prejudice, losing weight increases social acceptance and opens doors for better work opportunities, friendships, and even intimate relationships. Most people experience (with some occasional resentment) the favorable way that other people respond to their new shape, both socially and professionally.

Mobility and Comfort

Before surgery, physical activity may have been challenging and painful. Even walking may have been uncomfortable for you. After surgery, your physical options are virtually unlimited. Walking, biking, climbing, swimming, and participating in other physical activities are much easier and pain-free. You also may be able to squeeze into previously inconceivable spaces, such as restaurant booths and theater seats. And imagine not having to need that seat-belt extender!

Chapter 25

Ten Ways to Stay on the Straight and Narrow

. . . .

In This Chapter
▶ Keeping the weight off for life
▶ Committing to your success
▶ Being realistic about your goals

. . . .

*Y*our new stomach (whether it's banded, divided, or partially removed) will provide you with more self-control when it comes to food — at least for the first 12 to 18 months. What you choose to do with your newfound freedom is up to you. Your old habits need not apply.

In this chapter, we give you suggestions that will help keep you healthy and fit for life.

Plan Your Meals

You're more likely to stay with your new eating plan and less likely to go through the drive-thru if you plan your meals in advance. Packing your lunch the night before will save you time, money, and calories. Having dinner planned in advance with the appropriate healthy foods will help you resist making poor food choices.

Eat protein first. Keep healthy snacks on hand and junk food out of your house. Don't engage in other activities when you eat. Turn off the TV, don't talk on the phone, and put down the magazine.

Take your vitamins and supplements regularly. Doing so will ensure your body is properly nourished and help prevent any health problems related to deficiencies.

Keep a Food Log

A major step in successful weight loss is to become aware of when and how much you eat. You may discover that certain emotions trigger eating binges. Or you may snack your way through the day or do a lot of eating on the run. Keep track of when you eat or drink. This way you can make sure you're consuming the recommended protein, nutrients, and fluids throughout the day.

Free websites such as FitDay (www.fitday.com), Lose It! (www.loseit.com), and MyFitnessPal (www.myfitnesspal.com) can help you log your food and exercise. If you have a smartphone (such as an iPhone or Android), you can find apps for these sites, too.

Exercise

What you eat is only one part of the equation. Try to make physical activity a regular part of your day. Take it slow and steady. Start by walking, swimming, hiking, or doing any physical activity you enjoy. Find an exercise partner or class to help you stay interested. Exercise builds inner and outer strength. You'll also have more energy and feel less stress.

Mix up your routine every once in a while to keep it stimulating.

Join a Support Group

Attend support groups faithfully. The value of coming together with others in support groups and sharing your experiences and concerns is immeasurable. They allow you to see that you aren't alone in your struggles and challenges. They also give you an opportunity to give back to other patients, making their journey an easier ride.

You have to practice new behaviors in order to make them habits. Support groups are a good place to practice your new and healthy behaviors in a positive and supportive environment. You can attend in person or join an online support group.

Have a Buddy to Call in Times of Crisis

Reach out and call a friend for encouragement. This friend should be someone who will provide a positive influence and believes in you. Find someone or a few people you can rely on to help manage the stress and changes you'll be experiencing. They can be there to remind you how far you've come.

Remember That You're Worth It

You deserve the very best in life. You're allowed to be happy and live the life you want.

Take a few minutes throughout the day and imagine how you want to live your life. Visualize yourself happy, healthy, and energetic. You're feeling this way because you decided to make positive changes in your life, such as eating healthy foods, increasing your physical activity, and embracing self-love. Do this not because you *have* to but because you *want* to.

Stay in Touch with Your Surgeon

A unique patient-physician relationship exists in the weight loss surgery community. Most doctors' interest is greater than just the physical progress of their patients. They feel a personal satisfaction as *all* aspects of their patients' lives improve.

If you're experiencing any difficulty after surgery, give your doctor a call. Chances are, whatever the issue is, your doctor has seen it before and will be able to get you back on track.

Acknowledge and Commit

Keep the promise to yourself that you'll make this surgery work. Keep moving forward and take personal responsibility for your success. Commit to your new lifestyle and realize that you have to move it and shake it to keep the weight off. Commit to changing your eating habits; nothing in life is for free. Empower yourself to know that, if you want it, you can go out and achieve it.

Celebrate Your Success

Always acknowledge or celebrate any victory, no matter how big or small. (Just make sure you aren't using food as a reward!) Think about all the things you can do now that you couldn't do before. Keep a list of these things as a reminder and motivator (for example, the first time you could cross your legs, sit in a plane seat comfortably without the extender, or walk up a flight of stairs without becoming breathless). Achieving your emotional and psychological goals can be just as rewarding as losing the weight — if not more.

Be Realistic

Set hopeful but realistic expectations. Be flexible with your goals. The surgery won't solve all your problems. You'll lose weight, but everyone loses weight at his or her own rate and pace. Will you be one of the few who reaches the ideal body weight? Or will you lose 50 percent of your weight, feel better about yourself, and lose your obesity-related health problems?

Be patient with the process. Setbacks and disappointments are a part of the journey. If you have a slip, remember that you can get out of that rut and get back on track.

You'll hit plateaus and you may gain back some weight. This happens to most weight loss surgery patients. But realize that you can impact your weight loss with healthy food choices and increased activity. You can determine some, if not all, of your destiny.

Index

Apple & Mac

iPad 2 For Dummies,
3rd Edition
978-1-118-17679-5

iPhone 4S For Dummies,
5th Edition
978-1-118-03671-6

iPod touch For Dummies,
3rd Edition
978-1-118-12960-9

Mac OS X Lion
For Dummies
978-1-118-02205-4

Blogging & Social Media

CityVille For Dummies
978-1-118-08337-6

Facebook For Dummies,
4th Edition
978-1-118-09562-1

Mom Blogging
For Dummies
978-1-118-03843-7

Twitter For Dummies,
2nd Edition
978-0-470-76879-2

WordPress For Dummies,
4th Edition
978-1-118-07342-1

Business

Cash Flow For Dummies
978-1-118-01850-7

Investing For Dummies,
6th Edition
978-0-470-90545-6

Job Searching with Social
Media For Dummies
978-0-470-93072-4

QuickBooks 2012
For Dummies
978-1-118-09120-3

Resumes For Dummies,
6th Edition
978-0-470-87361-8

Starting an Etsy Business
For Dummies
978-0-470-93067-0

Cooking & Entertaining

Cooking Basics
For Dummies, 4th Edition
978-0-470-91388-8

Wine For Dummies,
4th Edition
978-0-470-04579-4

Diet & Nutrition

Kettlebells For Dummies
978-0-470-59929-7

Nutrition For Dummies,
5th Edition
978-0-470-93231-5

Restaurant Calorie Counter
For Dummies,
2nd Edition
978-0-470-64405-8

Digital Photography

Digital SLR Cameras &
Photography For Dummies,
4th Edition
978-1-118-14489-3

Digital SLR Settings
& Shortcuts
For Dummies
978-0-470-91763-3

Photoshop Elements 10
For Dummies
978-1-118-10742-3

Gardening

Gardening Basics
For Dummies
978-0-470-03749-2

Vegetable Gardening
For Dummies,
2nd Edition
978-0-470-49870-5

Green/Sustainable

Raising Chickens
For Dummies
978-0-470-46544-8

Green Cleaning
For Dummies
978-0-470-39106-8

Health

Diabetes For Dummies,
3rd Edition
978-0-470-27086-8

Food Allergies
For Dummies
978-0-470-09584-3

Living Gluten-Free
For Dummies,
2nd Edition
978-0-470-58589-4

Hobbies

Beekeeping
For Dummies,
2nd Edition
978-0-470-43065-1

Chess For Dummies,
3rd Edition
978-1-118-01695-4

Drawing For Dummies,
2nd Edition
978-0-470-61842-4

eBay For Dummies,
7th Edition
978-1-118-09806-6

Knitting For Dummies,
2nd Edition
978-0-470-28747-7

Language &
Foreign Language

English Grammar
For Dummies,
2nd Edition
978-0-470-54664-2

French For Dummies,
2nd Edition
978-1-118-00464-7

German For Dummies,
2nd Edition
978-0-470-90101-4

Spanish Essentials
For Dummies
978-0-470-63751-7

Spanish For Dummies,
2nd Edition
978-0-470-87855-2

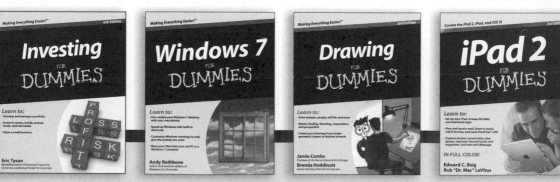

Math & Science

Algebra I For Dummies,
2nd Edition
978-0-470-55964-2

Biology For Dummies,
2nd Edition
978-0-470-59875-7

Chemistry For Dummies,
2nd Edition
978-1-1180-0730-3

Geometry For Dummies,
2nd Edition
978-0-470-08946-0

Pre-Algebra Essentials
For Dummies
978-0-470-61838-7

Microsoft Office

Excel 2010 For Dummies
978-0-470-48953-6

Office 2010 All-in-One
For Dummies
978-0-470-49748-7

Office 2011 for Mac
For Dummies
978-0-470-87869-9

Word 2010
For Dummies
978-0-470-48772-3

Music

Guitar For Dummies,
2nd Edition
978-0-7645-9904-0

Clarinet For Dummies
978-0-470-58477-4

iPod & iTunes
For Dummies,
9th Edition
978-1-118-13060-5

Pets

Cats For Dummies,
2nd Edition
978-0-7645-5275-5

Dogs All-in One
For Dummies
978-0470-52978-2

Saltwater Aquariums
For Dummies
978-0-470-06805-2

Religion & Inspiration

The Bible For Dummies
978-0-7645-5296-0

Catholicism For Dummies,
2nd Edition
978-1-118-07778-8

Spirituality For Dummies,
2nd Edition
978-0-470-19142-2

Self-Help & Relationships

Happiness For Dummies
978-0-470-28171-0

Overcoming Anxiety
For Dummies,
2nd Edition
978-0-470-57441-6

Seniors

Crosswords For Seniors
For Dummies
978-0-470-49157-7

iPad 2 For Seniors
For Dummies, 3rd Edition
978-1-118-17678-8

Laptops & Tablets
For Seniors For Dummies,
2nd Edition
978-1-118-09596-6

Smartphones & Tablets

BlackBerry For Dummies,
5th Edition
978-1-118-10035-6

Droid X2 For Dummies
978-1-118-14864-8

HTC ThunderBolt
For Dummies
978-1-118-07601-9

MOTOROLA XOOM
For Dummies
978-1-118-08835-7

Sports

Basketball For Dummies,
3rd Edition
978-1-118-07374-2

Football For Dummies,
2nd Edition
978-1-118-01261-1

Golf For Dummies,
4th Edition
978-0-470-88279-5

Test Prep

ACT For Dummies,
5th Edition
978-1-118-01259-8

ASVAB For Dummies,
3rd Edition
978-0-470-63760-9

The GRE Test For
Dummies, 7th Edition
978-0-470-00919-2

Police Officer Exam
For Dummies
978-0-470-88724-0

Series 7 Exam
For Dummies
978-0-470-09932-2

Web Development

HTML, CSS, & XHTML
For Dummies, 7th Edition
978-0-470-91659-9

Drupal For Dummies,
2nd Edition
978-1-118-08348-2

Windows 7

Windows 7
For Dummies
978-0-470-49743-2

Windows 7
For Dummies,
Book + DVD Bundle
978-0-470-52398-8

Windows 7 All-in-One
For Dummies
978-0-470-48763-1

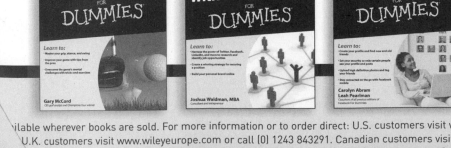

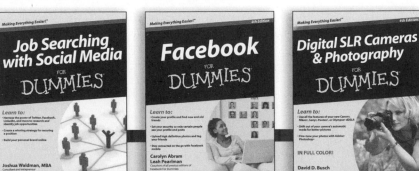